Impacts of Marine Corps Body Composition and Military Appearance Program (BCMAP) Standards on Individual Outcomes and Talent Management

JEANNETTE GAUDRY HAYNIE, JOSLYN FLEMING,
ALICIA REVITSKY LOCKER, ALICE SHIH

Prepared for the Navy and Marine Forces (NMF) Center
Approved for public release; distribution unlimited

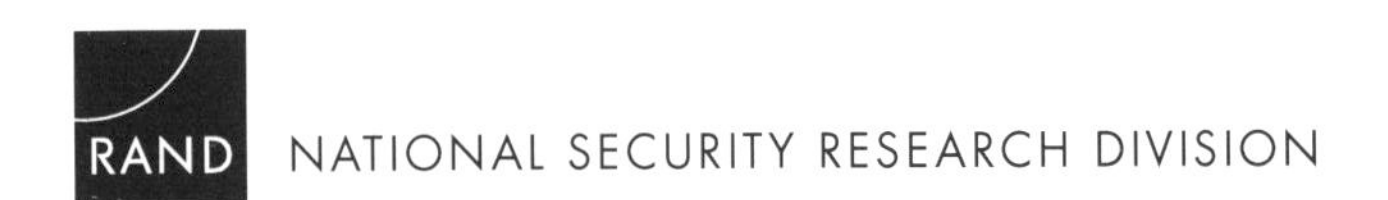

For more information on this publication, visit **www.rand.org/t/RRA1189-1**.

Published by the RAND Corporation, Santa Monica, Calif.

Library of Congress Cataloging-in-Publication Data is available for this publication.
ISBN: 978-1-9774-0881-5

Cover: Photo by Lance Cpl. David Bessey.

About This Report

Recent research conducted by military and academic scholars observed that the U.S. Marine Corps' Body Composition and Military Appearance Program (BCMAP) standards were not developed from populations that reflect the current makeup of the force and the fitness requirements that they are subject to. Research findings suggest that the implementation of these standards could drive marines to adopt unhealthy behaviors, primarily those associated with disordered eating, to meet the standards while disproportionately affecting communities of color and women more generally. Furthermore, these unhealthy behaviors can cause significant short- and long-term mental and physical health problems that could negatively affect individual marines during their service and long after. Although there is some limited research on body-composition standards and eating disorders in the services, there has been little assessment of how the negative effects of policy and the behaviors associated with it affect the mental and physical health of individual marines (particularly those from communities of color and women more generally), career retention, and overall military readiness. Service and U.S. Department of Defense leadership have made talent management and diversity of the force at different levels of leadership an institutional priority; therefore, understanding how the BCMAP is affecting the force will help meet these objectives.

This report will help decisionmakers understand how the BCMAP and its associated policies drive individual behavior, particularly for women in general and communities of color. It will also inform talent-management efforts and discussions about relevant national security implications while providing recommendations and a general framework for policy change. Building awareness of current research in healthy body standards and relevant characteristics—and identifying any gaps between existing policy and current research—could inform more-effective policy development.

RAND National Security Research Division

This research was sponsored by the Office of the Secretary of Defense and conducted within the Navy and Marine Forces (NMF) Center of the RAND National Security Research Division (NSRD), which operates the RAND National Defense Research Institute (NDRI), a federally funded research and development center sponsored by the Office of the Secretary of Defense, the Joint Staff, the Unified Combatant Commands, the Navy, the Marine Corps, the defense agencies, and the defense intelligence enterprise.

For more information on the RAND NMF Center, see www.rand.org/nsrd/nmf or contact the director (contact information is provided on the webpage).

Acknowledgments

We would like to express immense gratitude to RAND NMF Center leadership, Paul DeLuca and Brendan Toland, for their support of this research project. We would also like to thank our peer reviewers, Molly McIntosh and Kyleanne Hunter.

Summary

The authors of this report present the findings from an initial scoping analysis of the individual and institutional impacts of the current U.S. Marine Corps' Body Composition and Military Appearance Program (BCMAP), offer recommendations for immediate actions and additional research, and provide a framework to support policy change.

Issue

Marine Corps body-composition standards and associated policies may be encouraging behaviors that could cause long-term harm to both marines and the force. Research indicates that the BCMAP was developed using outdated data that do not reflect the diverse makeup of the current force or the physical fitness standards that marines must meet.[1] This can affect the Marine Corps' ability to retain the ready force it seeks to cultivate while placing marines at risk of adopting unhealthy behaviors that could have long-lasting impacts on their health.[2] Our research seeks to understand two fundamental questions:

1. What is the existing policy, and what are its scientific foundations?
2. What are the possible impacts of the policy, either clear or hidden, on the individual marine and the overall Marine Corps organization?

---

[1] Kerry Hogan, *Review of the Current Body Fat Taping Method and Its Importance in Ascertaining Fitness Levels in the United States Marine Corps*, dissertation, Monterey, Calif.: Naval Postgraduate School, 2015.

[2] Existing research includes Ulla Kärkkäinen, Linda Mustelin, Anu Raevuori, Jaakko Kaprio, and Anna Keski-Rahkonen, "Do Disordered Eating Behaviours Have Long-Term Health-Related Consequences?" *European Eating Disorders Review*, Vol. 26, No. 1, January 2018; Peggy Anne Fisher McNulty, "Prevalence and Contributing Factors of Eating Disorder Behaviors in Active Duty Service Women in the Army, Navy, Air Force, and Marines," *Military Medicine*, Vol. 166, No. 1, January 2001; and Katie M. O'Brien, Denis R. Whelan, Dale P. Sandler, Janet E. Hall, and Clarice R. Weinberg, "Predictors and Long-Term Health Outcomes of Eating Disorders," *PLOS One*, Vol. 12, No. 7, July 2017.

Approach

We approached our research questions with a research review drawing on publicly available reporting about body-composition standards and their associated impacts. We focused our review on four key research subject areas: (1) existing policy and its scientific foundations, (2) the impact of body-composition standards on individual health choices, (3) the impacts of these health choices on the short- and long-term mental and physical health of personnel, and (4) the impacts on the Marine Corps (including retention and diversity, equity, and inclusion efforts). We used qualitative data-analysis tools to conduct a thematic analysis of the literature and then group findings by topic area. Using this research, we propose recommendations for immediate actions and future research and outline a framework to provide a variety of policy options for Marine Corps leadership to consider in the future.

Assumptions and Limitations

Initiated by the RAND Corporation, this research project aims to address a timely topic in the military policy domain. This research was exploratory and relied on existing literature. We did not conduct interviews or collect data collection because of funding provisions.

Our review of the evidentiary base identified that the literature related specifically to the Marine Corps' body-composition policy and its associated impacts was relatively sparse, with limited sources dated after 2015.[3]

[3] The primary references with Marine Corps–specific data included Hogan, 2015; McNulty, 2001; Armed Forces Health Surveillance Center, "Diagnoses of Overweight/Obesity, Active Component, U.S. Armed Forces, 1998–2010," *Medical Surveillance Monthly Report*, Vol. 18, No. 1, January 2008; Institute of Medicine, *Assessing Readiness in Military Women: The Relationship of Body, Composition, Nutrition, and Health*, Washington, D.C.: National Academies Press, 1998; Crescent A. Seibert, *Demographic, Psychological, and Weight-Related Correlates of Weight Control Behaviors Among Active Duty Military Personnel*, thesis, Bethesda, Md.: Uniformed Services University of the Health Sciences, March 2007; Sharon Silas, *Department of Defense: Eating Disorders in the Military*, Washington, D.C.: U.S. Government Accountability Office, GAO-20-611R, August 7, 2020; Defense Health Board, *Implications of Trends in Obesity and Overweight for the Department of Defense*, Falls Church, Va., November 22, 2013.

However, the evidentiary base related more broadly to body composition in the U.S. Department of Defense (DoD) and literature focused on similar groups (veterans, athletes) were much more comprehensive and current. Drawing on this larger evidentiary base, we present our findings and recommendations.

Despite the sparse evidentiary base of literature pertaining specifically to the Marine Corps, the significant and recent media reporting surrounding the issue—and efforts by the Marine Corps' Women's Initiative Team (WIT)[4] to bring attention to the topic and have this policy examined and discussed at senior leadership levels—indicate that the Marine Corps and other services are affected by this issue.[5]

Key Findings

We found that the Marine Corps' emphasis on strict adherence to fitness standards and the importance of physical appearance as a quality necessary to lead marines are two issues that amplify each other. This may drive marines to adopt unhealthy behaviors to conform to standards outlined in the BCMAP. The implementation of the policy likely causes unintended consequences that are at odds with its stated purpose.

Furthermore, we observed the following key findings related to BCMAP and its impact on the force:

---

[4] WIT is a grassroots organization that uses social media, specifically Facebook and podcasts, to connect female marines and marine allies on issues that significantly impact women. The Air Force also has an established WIT, and the teams have worked together to cover such topics as body composition and maternity uniforms (see, for example, Gina Harkins, "Female Marines Who Called Out the Corps Commend New Postpartum Policy," *Military.com*, February 11, 2021).

[5] Recent media articles about this include Haley Britzky, "'We Are All Suffering in Silence'—Inside the US Military's Pervasive Culture of Eating Disorders," *Task and Purpose*, August 2, 2021; Oriana Pawlyk, "Air Force Becomes First Service to Ditch the Hated Tape Test for Good," *Military.com*, December 8, 2020; and Sharon Sisbarro, Kerry Hogan, Sara Kirstein, and Catherine Baniakas, "The DoD's Body Composition Standards Are Harming Female Service Members," *Military.com*, December 31, 2020.

- **Changes to the BCMAP over the decades have been incremental.** Although the Marine Corps may have developed a better understanding of the issue, it still needs to examine the policy more holistically to determine how changes could fundamentally affect both individuals and the force.
- **Relatedly, physical fitness requirements have increased for all marines, but revisions to the BCMAP have not sufficiently accounted for these changes.** Today's fitness standards, particularly for those ground combat military occupational specialties (MOSs) that were recently opened to women, require that marines build muscle mass, which can lead to increased weight. Although the BCMAP has been revised as recently as 2021, to account for these new requirements, revisions do not appear to sufficiently account for these increased fitness requirements.
- **Height and weight tables are drawn from unrepresentative populations and may disproportionately affect people of color and women, particularly women of color.** This may have impacts on the health and retention of the force.
- **To meet standards, marines are adopting unhealthy eating disorder behaviors; diagnosis rates for such disorders may be underreported.** Marines are diagnosed with eating disorders at higher rates than other service members, and women marines in particular are diagnosed more than others. The stigma and hidden nature of eating disorders often mean that not everyone who shows symptoms is diagnosed. Risky behaviors can include self-induced vomiting, laxative and diet pill use, sauna and diuretic use, excessive exercise, and fasting. Existing research notes the significantly elevated rates of these behaviors among service members, including the limited research of marine behavior. Additionally, service members have seen associated short- and long-term mental and physical health impacts, including cognitive functioning impairment, reproductive and skeletal problems, depression, and suicide risk.
- **This is an understudied problem; more research is needed to understand the full breadth of impacts.** Areas identified as lacking significant study include retention (particularly for women and

especially women of color), impact on the health choices and retention of pregnant and postpartum women, and impacts on readiness.

Recommendations

We make the following recommendations based on our research:

- The Marine Corps should take a comprehensive, systematic approach to fully understand and address the deficiencies in the BCMAP, develop a more health-focused policy, and mitigate any impacts from the existing BCMAP through research and analysis. This approach should clearly define the objective of the policy; thoroughly investigate possible alternatives for feasibility, risk, and cost; compare alternatives in terms of outcomes; and assess and mitigate any potential negative impacts of the existing BCMAP.
- For the safety of all marines and the health of the force, we recommend pausing all height, weight, and body-composition measurements as additional recommendations are considered.
- Reevaluate whether height, weight, and body-composition measurements are still necessary for marines and whether those measurements are as representative of overall fitness and health as the BCMAP considers them to be, especially for marines from specific demographic groups and in the context of specific MOS requirements.
- Reassess the need to include verbiage in the BCMAP that directly links weight and appearance to the leadership, discipline, and character of marines. Although appearance is an important functional part of Marine Corps culture, the emphasis to "make weight" can result in unhealthy behaviors and lead to shame. We recommend that the Marine Corps clarify and balance out this tension.
- Develop and implement a body-composition program that directly grapples with the contradictory nature of the existing program; create a new program that delineates requirements both for health and performance and that includes requirements designed to reflect and support the diversity of the force.

Finally, we found to be problematic the absence of substantive research about how all groups are potentially affected by the BCMAP, existing standards and measurement methods, and disordered eating behavior. We view our recommendations as first steps, and we recommend additional research into how service members across DoD are affected by DoD and service policies, how veterans are affected by longer-term disordered eating behaviors and associated mental and physical health comorbidities, and how these factors may influence retention and readiness as a whole across DoD.

We recommend the following to extend research efforts on the topic:

- Conduct an analysis to understand who may be on the cusp of failing standards and therefore may be more at risk for harmful behaviors. This analysis should also include a broader survey or analysis of a large marine population, particularly those of myriad demographic groups.
- Broadly collect and analyze data. From the first recommendation—screening and analysis to reach out to the Marine Corps veteran community—a broader analysis of those potentially affected by the BCMAP and how such manifestations could identify individuals who are still at risk of harm today. This data collection and analysis should also include transgender marines, namely to identify how binary gender standards may affect them and what healthy standards could be.
- Assess whether and how Marine Corps culture may have coalesced around the existing BCMAP. Cultures that emphasize appearance and weight can place members at increased risk for unhealthy behavior. A clear education and communication strategy may be needed to ensure that culture changes accompany policy shifts.
- Understand the totality of the issue by including more research into why service members leave the force and if their decisions are influenced by the BCMAP.
- Conduct more research that explores the impact of the body-composition policy on military readiness and the lethality of the force.

Contents

Figures and Tables

Figures

Tables

CHAPTER ONE

Introduction

Recent media reporting has drawn attention to the fact that the U.S. Marine Corps' Body Composition and Military Appearance Policy (BCMAP) standards may be outdated.[1] These dated standards could negatively affect the health of individual marines, the health of the force, Marine Corps talent-management efforts, the diversity of the force, and overall military readiness.[2] The BCMAP aims to ensure that marines comply with established body-composition standards and present a "suitable military appearance,"[3] while conforming to physical fitness standards. However, the BCMAP standards as they are measured and applied use outdated data from 1984 and were developed by researching subjects that do not reflect the current Marine Corps population. Recent reporting indicates that these standards and their measures overpredict body fat and disproportionately affect certain ethnic groups (Hispanic, African American) and women in general,

[1] Central to our research questions are standards for the weight-height and body fat standards that are the focus of the BCMAP. It does not include physical fitness standards or military occupational specialty standards (MOSs) that are codified in other Marine Corps policies. The BCMAP is separate from the Marine Corps Physical Fitness Program (MCPFP), but the MCPFP and BCMAP are combined to form a comprehensive program. We provide a more extended explanation of these three different types of standards—weight-height and body fat standards, Marine Corps physical fitness standards, and MOSs—in the next chapter.

[2] Sharon Sisbarro, Kerry Hogan, Sara Kirstein, and Catherine Baniakas, "The DoD's Body Composition Standards Are Harming Female Service Members," *Military.com*, December 31, 2020.

[3] Marine Corps Order (MCO) 6110.3A CH-1 and Admin CH, *Marine Corps Body Composition and Military Appearance Program*, Washington, D.C.: Department of the Navy, Headquarters United States Marine Corps, April 16, 2019, p. 2.

potentially negatively affecting marines in a various ways. Additionally, as the physical fitness demands on the force have changed to meet warfighting demands, the policies for body composition have stayed mostly static.

The emphasis placed on these standards may compel marines, and specifically female marines, to adopt unhealthy behaviors to comply with the policy in order to be competitive for promotion, command, and retention. Female marines are diagnosed with eating disorders at higher rates than any other group in the U.S. Department of Defense (DoD), and eating disorder behavior can have long-term negative mental and physical health outcomes for marines who experience it, including low bone mass, amenorrhea and reproductive health problems, anxiety, and depression.[4] Current application of the BCMAP and estimates of its impacts may not be capturing the full extent of the issues the force faces because of the sensitive nature of these topics.

Although there has been considerable research about the impacts of DoD standards on recruitment, fitness, and task performance,[5] little research has been done to assess impacts of established standards on individual health choices and the health of the force, talent management and career retention, the diversity of the force, and overall military readiness.[6] Therefore, this report focuses on understanding the research space with regard to Marine

---

[4] Hubertus Himmerich, Carol Kan, Katie Au, and Janet Treasure, "Pharmacological Treatment of Eating Disorders, Comorbid Mental Health Problems, Malnutrition, and Physical Health Consequences," *Pharmacology and Therapeutics*, Vol. 217, January 2021; and Peggy Anne Fisher McNulty, "Prevalence and Contributing Factors of Eating Disorder Behaviors in Active Duty Service Women in the Army, Navy, Air Force, and Marines," *Military Medicine*, Vol. 166, No. 1, January 2001.

[5] This is exemplified in Defense Health Board, "Implications of Trends in Obesity and Overweight for the Department of Defense," Falls Church, Va., November 22, 2013; and Institute of Medicine, *Assessing Readiness in Military Women: The Relationship of Body, Composition, Nutrition, and Health*, Washington, D.C.: National Academies Press, 1998.

[6] Additionally, there have been efforts to look at this from a DoD-wide but not from a service-specific perspective. As part of its 2019 report, the Defense Advisory Committee on Women in the Services investigated DoD policy related to body composition and made recommendations to conduct a comprehensive review of body weight standards and measurement techniques (see Defense Advisory Committee on Women in the Services, *2019 Annual Report*, November 13, 2019).

Corps body-composition standards, measurements, and overall impacts. Understanding the standards and policy impacts can provide policymakers with tangible solutions to address deficiencies in current policies, provide care for service members, and increase the overall readiness and performance of the force.

To conduct our research review, we drew on publicly available reporting pertaining to body-composition standards and associated impacts. We derived our definition of *body composition* from military service policies.[7] From the definition, we created search parameters to understand the issue across four key research subject areas: (1) existing policy and the scientific foundations for associated body-composition standards, (2) impacts of body-composition standards on individual health choices, (3) impacts of health choices on marines' short- and long-term health, and (4) impacts on retention of military personnel. Once search parameters were set, we analyzed the literature and group findings by topic area. The volume of research in this area is extensive and diverse; therefore, the review of literature was broad but not complete. We asked the following questions for each of the four key research subject areas:

- **Existing policy and scientific foundations for standards:** What is the existing Marine Corps policy, and what is the science behind it? What does the literature say about potential measurement standards? How has the science changed?
- **Impacts on individual health choices:** What are the research-supported impacts and hypothesized impacts of body-composition policies on an individual marine's health choices? What are the behavior patterns associated with these health choices?
- **Impacts of health choices on mental and physical health:** What are the impacts of these health choices on the short- and long-term mental and physical health of personnel? Do these have potential impacts on cognitive function and decisionmaking?

[7] Body composition consists of two major elements of the human body: lean body mass (including muscle, bone, and essential organ tissue) and body fat (Army Regulation 600-9, *The Army Weight Control Program*, Washington, D.C.: Headquarters, Department of the Army, November 27, 2006).

- **Impacts to the institution:** How do the policies impact a marine's decision to retain or separate? What are the impacts to retaining a lethal and diverse force? What impacts do the policies have on marines of different genders, races, or ethnicities? Do these impacts shape retention of marines across different genders, races, or ethnicities?

Impacts on pregnant and postpartum women and the unique challenges that they face upon returning to duty were beyond the scope of this project. Additionally, although potential impacts on readiness were beyond the scope of the study, readiness implications were considered and identified when appropriate.

The review also highlighted understudied or overlooked topics related to body-composition standards and their impacts. Our research led us to propose recommendations for action, future research, and creating a framework to provide a variety of policy options for Marine Corps leadership to consider in the future.

Assumptions and Limitations

Initiated by the RAND Corporation, this research project aims to address a timely topic within the military policy domain. This research was exploratory and relied on existing literature. We did not conduct interviews or collect data because of funding provisions.

Our review of the evidentiary base identified that the literature related specifically to the Marine Corps' body-composition policy and its associated impacts was relatively sparse, with limited sources dated after 2015.[8]

[8] The primary references with Marine Corps–specific data included Kerry Hogan, *Review of the Current Body Fat Taping Method and Its Importance in Ascertaining Fitness Levels in the United States Marine Corps*, dissertation, Monterey, Calif.: Naval Postgraduate School, 2015; McNulty, 2001; Armed Forces Health Surveillance Center, "Diagnoses of Overweight/Obesity, Active Component, U.S. Armed Forces, 1998–2010," *Medical Surveillance Monthly Report*, Vol. 18, No. 1, January 2008; Institute of Medicine, 1998; Crescent A. Seibert, *Demographic, Psychological, and Weight-Related Correlates of Weight Control Behaviors Among Active Duty Military Personnel*, thesis, Bethesda, Md.: Uniformed Services University of the Health Sciences, March 2007; Sharon Silas, *Department of Defense: Eating Disorders in the Military*, Washington,

However, the evidentiary base related more broadly to body composition in DoD and literature focused on similar groups (veterans, athletes) were much more comprehensive and current. This broader evidentiary base informed our findings and recommendations.

Despite the sparse evidentiary base of literature pertaining specifically to the Marine Corps, the significant and recent media reporting surrounding the issue—and efforts by the Marine Corps' Women's Initiative Team (WIT)[9] to bring attention to the topic and have this policy examined and discussed at senior leadership levels—indicate that the Marine Corps and other services are affected by this issue.[10]

D.C.: U.S. Government Accountability Office, GAO-20-611R, August 7, 2020; Defense Health Board, 2013.

[9] WIT is a grassroots organization that uses via social media, specifically Facebook and podcasts, to connect female marines and marine allies on issues that significantly impact women. The Air Force also has an established WIT, and the teams have worked together to cover such topics as body composition and maternity uniforms (see, for example, Gina Harkins, "Female Marines Who Called Out the Corps Commend New Postpartum Policy," *Military.com*, February 11, 2021).

[10] A sample of recent media articles include Oriana Pawlyk, "Air Force Becomes First Service to Ditch the Hated Tape Test for Good," *Military.com*, December 8, 2020; Sisbarro et al., 2020; and Haley Britzky, "'We Are All Suffering in Silence'—Inside the US Military's Pervasive Culture of Eating Disorders," *Task and Purpose*, August 2, 2021.

CHAPTER TWO

Evolution of Body Composition Standards in the Marine Corps

Height and weight standards for the military services have evolved since the Marine Corps' inception to reflect national trends on ideal body-composition standards. Although the overall goal of height and weight standards has been to produce a service member who is "fit to fight," that definition has changed over the years. Thus, the Marine Corps has incrementally changed its standards to balance the need to address concerns about rising obesity trends and the need to design standards that match changes in fitness requirements. As the needs of the military change, these standards continue to evolve. Although a single DoD standard has been in place since 1981, each service has implemented slightly different body-composition policies to reflect their respective needs. Understanding the evolution of the BCMAP and how it relates to the other services is helpful in providing a basis of understanding for the research questions explored in this report.

Current Body Composition Definition and Scope

Department of Defense Instruction (DoDI) 1308.3, *DoD Physical Fitness and Body Fat Programs Procedures*,[1] provides overarching guidance on physical fitness, height/weight, and body-composition standards for the armed services. The instruction leaves development and implementation

[1] Department of Defense Instruction 1308.3, *DoD Physical Fitness and Body Fat Programs Procedures*, Washington, D.C.: U.S. Department of Defense, November 5, 2002.

of fitness and body-composition programs (BCPs) to each service. This allows each to develop standards that meet their specific needs and missions. Service programs must, at a minimum, meet the standards set by DoDI 1308.3, may not be more stringent than the body mass index (BMI[2]) tables prescribed in the instruction, and must use the circumference-based method of measurement to assess body fat. Guidance for the BCMAP is promulgated in MCO 6110.3A, established in 2016 and revised three times since.[3] The order lacks a standard definition of *body composition*, but the objective of the program is "to establish healthy weight and body-composition standards, and to ensure all marines present a suitable military appearance."[4] Therefore, the inference is that body composition relates specifically to height and weight standards and military appearance. The BCMAP is separate from the MCPFP, but the MCPFP and BCMAP are combined to form a comprehensive program to "enhance Marine wellness, body composition, and military appearance while diminishing other risk factors to improve Marine combat readiness and personal appearance."[5]

In accordance with MCO 6110.3A, height and weight measurements are a semiannual and annual requirement for all active-duty marines and reservists, respectively. Commanders are authorized to conduct weigh-ins or body-composition and military-appearance assessments as frequently as they deem necessary. Weigh-ins may be conducted on the same day as physical fitness assessments (PFAs). Equipment for the height and weight assessment consists of a non-stretching fiberglass tape measure attached to

---

[2] BMI is a widely used index developed to capture nutritional status and relative weight. The formula is weight in kilograms divided by height in meters (squared), and, per the Centers for Disease Control and Prevention (CDC), it represents "an inexpensive and easy screening method for weight category—underweight, healthy weight, overweight, and obesity" (Centers for Disease Control and Prevention, "About Adult BMI," webpage, August 27, 2021).

[3] MCO 6110.3A CH-1 and Admin CH occurred in October 2017 to provide amplifying guidance on medical exemption processes. MCO 6110.3A CH-2 occurred in April 2019 to revise pregnancy and post-pregnancy policy. MCO 6110.13A CH-3 occurred in February 2021 to further revise the pregnancy and post-pregnancy aspects of the policy (see MCO 6100.13A CH-3, 2021).

[4] MCO 6110.3A CH-1 and Admin CH, 2019, p. 1-1.

[5] MCO 6110.3A CH-1 and Admin CH, 2019, p. 2.

a vertical surface (e.g., the wall) and a calibrated digital or balance-beam scale. Height and weight measurements are cross-referenced with height and weight tables (see appendix).

If a marine fails to meet the authorized weight for height, a body-composition assessment (BCA) is required. The Marine Corps was the first of the services to institute a circumference-based measurement for estimating body fat. Body composition is estimated using the circumference-based method. According to the order, for male marines, this consists of measuring neck and abdominal circumference (at the navel). The circumference value is calculated by subtracting the neck from the abdominal measurement. For female marines, the neck, abdomen (thinnest part), and hips are measured. The calculation for circumference value is equal to adding the waist and hip measurements and subtracting the neck measurement. Circumference is measured using a self-tensioning taping device. Body circumference values are then compared with height tables to estimate body-fat percentages. Marines who exceed the body-fat standard are then referred to a BCP but only after receiving a medical evaluation. Marines referred to the BCP are subject to the administrative actions summarized in Table 2.1.

The Marine Corps allows certain waivers to the program based on extraordinary capability. Marines who score 285 and higher on both the Marine Corps Physical Fitness Test (PFT) and Marine Corps Combat Fitness Test (CFT) are exempt from maximum body weight percentages; however, their height, weight, and body fat are still recorded and reported.

Marines who score 250 and higher on both fitness tests are allowed an additional 1-percent body-fat limit. Commanders also have the authority to submit BCP assignment waivers for marines who exceed standards but present a suitable military appearance. The order emphasizes that this waiver should be reserved for the "rare" marine. Figure 2.1 summarizes the BCMAP process.

As of this writing, the Marine Corps has begun a formal study of the existing body-composition standards and methods in the context of individual performance capabilities. The study involves measuring volunteers' body composition via a three-dimensional body surface scan, a dual-energy X-ray absorptiometry scan, a bioelectrical impedance analysis, and a measurement of explosive lower body power. Testing started at Marine

TABLE 2.1
Administrative Actions After Body-Composition Program Assignment

Administrative Action After Body Composition Program (BCP) Assignment	1st	2nd
Mandatory remedial conditioning	Yes	Yes
Page 11 counseling entry (NAVMC 10274)[a]	Yes*	Yes*
Adverse fitness report (and mandatory section I comment)[b]	Yes	Yes
Substandard conduct marks	Yes	Yes
Promotion restriction	Yes	Yes
Eligible for permanent change of station/permanent change of assignment transfer	Yes	No
Eligible for reenlistment	No	No
Eligible for special school assignment	No	No
Process for administrative separation	Yes	Yes

SOURCE: MCO 6110.3A CH-1 and Admin CH, 2019, p. 1-16; small edits were made for capitalization and to remove abbreviations that do not appear in the rest of our report.
* Page 11 counseling entry is completed for initial assignment to BCP, follow-on entries are completed if marine fails to make adequate progress during the program.
[a] Page 11 counseling refers to an administrative mark in a marine's service record.
[b] Section I refers to the portion of a marine's fitness report for directed and additional comments—assignment to BCP requires mandatory language to be included in this section.

Corps Base Quantico but will shift to an unknown number of locations in the future. The Marine Corps is seeking 600–800 volunteers between the study's launch in June 2021 and its close in March 2022.[6] Although assessing the body-composition standards and methods is one element of our recommendations, we found that the potential impacts of the existing policy and associated standards potentially call for a more holistic response.

Evolution of Standards

The development of a DoD body-composition standard was established in 1981 with DoD Directive 1308.1, which established a body fat standard.

[6] Hope Hodge Seck, "Volunteer Testing Begins in Marines' Groundbreaking Body Composition Study," *Military.com*, June 10, 2021.

FIGURE 2.1

Marine Corps BCMAP Sequence Chart

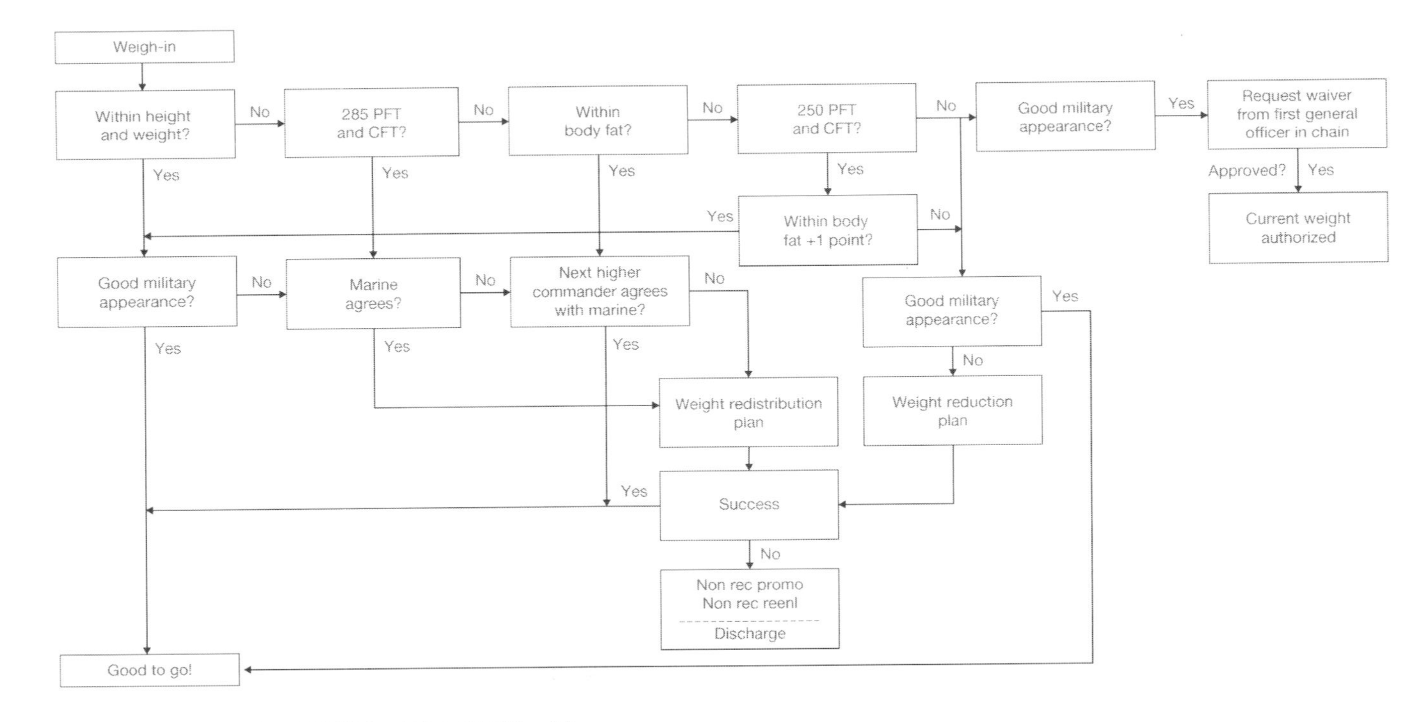

SOURCE: Adapted from MCO 6110.3A CH-1` and Admin CH, 2019, p. 2-1.
NOTES: Non rec promo = promotion not recommended; non rec reenl = reenlistment not recommended.

Prior to 1981, DoD—and the Marine Corps more specifically—had created standards to meet the needs of the force at the time. This included meeting minimum standards when malnourishment and disease were a concern and later minimum and maximum requirements for heights and weights when national concern over obesity in the force became a concern. Table 2.2 provides a synopsis of the evolution of these standards and provides historical context for the changes in guidance and policy.

Historically, height and weight standards in the Marine Corps were developed to keep *underweight men* from weakening units, because being underweight was associated with a less healthy and fit life. These were primarily minimum and not maximum standards; therefore, because of existing roles in the service, women were not the focus—men were.[7] As the makeup of the force changed to include a more diverse population, so too did the Marine Corps' body-composition standards change. Beginning in 1945, the Marine Corps started to include body-composition metrics for women. The role of women in the Marine Corps has changed significantly since. Major changes include women's continued service during and after pregnancy, the rescission of the ground combat exclusion policy, and changes to PFAs, which require more strength.

Inclusion of women and the expansion of their roles are not the only factors that have spurred change in the Marine Corps' body-composition policy. The increase in obesity in the general U.S. population has raised concerns that the military population is also gaining weight. Between the 1980s and the present, the Marine Corps has periodically changed the standards to address concerns over the rise in obesity, while also answering demands by Congress to ensure that the standards are not overly restrictive or negatively affect the careers of marines who belong to specific populations.

In addition to changes to the BCMAP, the Marine Corps has evolved its physical fitness requirements to meet the demands of a more lethal, deployable force. With these increased requirements, including job-specific standards for specifically coded MOSs, the Marine Corps' emphasis within the BCMAP on lean and trim is at odds with the physical capabilities it demands of its force.

---

[7] Hogan, 2015.

TABLE 2.2

Evolution of Marine Corps Body Composition Standards with Historical Context

Period	Significant Change in Policy	Reason/Context for Change in Guidance or Policy	Maximum Body Fat Percentage	Marine Corps Policy
1865–1945	Established minimum standards	To be deemed "fit to fight," minimum standards ensured that volunteers were not malnourished or had diseases.	N/A	No specific policy number
1945	Established minimum standards for women and an "ideal" weight standard (no maximum)	Healthy weights were emphasized based on statistics from life insurance companies regarding shortened life expectancy for obese individuals.	N/A	MCO 6100.3C[a]
1968	Established minimum and maximum heights for men, women, aviators, officers, enlisted; maximum weights further delineated by age group	There is no context.	N/A	MCO 6100.3C
1975	Revision of previous standards to eliminate age group categories and specific height for weights for specific MOSs (e.g. aviators)	There was an emphasis on physical fitness for *all* marines to ensure combat effectiveness regardless of age or duty assignment.	W: 23.3 M: 27.5	MCO 6100.3G[b]
1981	Addition of body fat standard	Changes were implemented after the release of President Carter's commissioned study, *Study of the Military Services Physical Fitness*,[c] because of public concern over an "overweight military."	W: 23.3 M: 27.5	DoD Directive 1308.1; DoDI 1308.3

TABLE 2.2—CONTINUED

Period	Significant Change in Policy	Reason/Context for Change in Guidance or Policy	Maximum Body Fat Percentage	Marine Corps Policy
1997	Inclusion of a body fat measurement for failure of height/weight standard instead of an alternate weight standard; measurements to calculate body weight for women were changed to use neck, waist and hips vice neck, forearm, thigh, biceps, and abdomen	Change in PFT standards, including different sit-ups, requirement for those over age 46 to test, and altitude variation added to the scoring tables. Marine Corps leadership indicated need for change was because of "performance being the key."	W: 23.3 M: 27.5	MCO 6100.10A[d]
2002	Increase in maximum body fat percentage for women to 25 percent; added performance exemption for first-class PFT	Increase for body fat percentage for women was in response to a U.S. Government Accounting Office report to the U.S. Senate articulating concerns about variability in body fat estimates across the services and its impact on women.	W: 25 M: 27.5	MCO 6100.3C[e]; DoDI 1308.3
2008	Severed link between physical fitness and personal appearance, inserted commander's assessment into evaluation of personal appearance; performance exemption rescinded	There was a response to a perceived trend of society being overweight.	W: 25 M: 27.5	MCO 6110.3[f]

TABLE 2.2—CONTINUED

Period	Significant Change in Policy	Reason/Context for Change in Guidance or Policy	Maximum Body Fat Percentage	Marine Corps Policy
2017	Modified maximum allowance for women to 26 percent; increased number of age categories to eight; use of self-tensioning measurement devices for more-precise measurement; decentralized BCP waiver-granting authority; BCP waiver for those who score a 285 or higher on fitness tests	There was a comprehensive review by Training and Education Command because of complaints that muscular marines were failing BCP tests; change in fitness requirements included modification of PFT/CFT tables and elimination of flex arm hang for women and requirement to do pull-ups or push-ups.	W: 26 M: 27.5	MCO 6110.3A

[a] Marine Corps Order 6100.3C, *Physical Fitness*, Washington, D.C.: Commandant of the Marine Corps, August 9, 1956.
[b] Marine Corps Order 6100.3G, *Physical Fitness, Weight Control and Military Appearance*, enclosure 1, Washington, D.C.: Commandant of the Marine Corps, September 23, 1975.
[c] U.S. Department of Defense, *Study of the Military Services Physical Fitness*, Washington, D.C., April 3, 1981.
[d] Marine Corps Order 6100.10A, *Weight Control and Military Appearance*, enclosures 2 and 3, Washington, D.C.: Commandant of the Marine Corps, May 10, 1986.
[e] Marine Corps Order P6100.12, *Marine Corps Physical Fitness Test and Body Composition Program Manual*, Washington, D.C.: Commandant of the Marine Corps, May 10, 2002.
[f] Marine Corps Order 6110.3, *Marine Corps Body Composition and Military Appearance Program*, Washington, D.C.: Commandant of the Marine Corps, August 8, 2008.

Evolution in Fitness Standards in the Marine Corps

Although the Marine Corps has separated the BCMAP from its fitness policy, the two are still linked. The MCPFP and the BCMAP are intended by the service to be a comprehensive program that ensures the overall health, readiness, and appearance of a marine.[8] Therefore, an understanding of the

[8] Per MCO 6110.3A CH-1 and Admin CH, 2019, p. 2:

> Combined with the Marine Corps Physical Fitness Program (MCPFP) contained in reference (b) and in recognition that Marines are warrior athletes, it is essential the Marine Corps develops a comprehensive program that will enhance Marine well-

evolution of the Marine Corps fitness standards provides context for why there have been changes in the BCMAP since its inception.

Between the 1960s and 2002, Marine Corps fitness standards and height/weight standards were revised three times—increasing from such activities as a shuttle run, broad jump, and a duck waddle to a three-mile run, crunches, and pull-ups for men and women, with some moderations, that still exist. But today's standards for men and women started at a significant distance apart. Fitness standards for men were set starting in the 1960s, with a series of exercises that involved body strength and some endurance. Older marines were initially exempted, and women were advised at the time to perform such exercises as a twist, leg raise, and hip roll. In fact, in 1963, the service published a pamphlet, "Slim and Trim: For Women Marines," that emphasized, "Women Marines must always be the smallest group of women in the military service. In accordance with the Commandant's desire, they must also be the most attractive and useful women in the four line services."[9] Women's fitness standards did not develop into more targeted exercises until the mid-1970s. At that time, height/weight standards for both men and women continued to emphasize minimums and ideals instead of maximums.[10]

In the mid-1990s, the Marine Corps PFT began to resemble its current incarnation, with men and women alike required to perform crunches and a three-mile run, pull-ups for men, and the flexed arm hang for women. In 2012, the service again changed the PFT to encourage women to similarly perform pull-ups, a standard that is still being refined today—with push-ups as an alternative.[11] In addition to PFT changes, in 2008, the Marine Corps launched the CFT as a complement to the PFT. The CFT is designed, per MCO 6100.13A with change 3 (February 2021), to measure general functional fitness and related skills. The CFT includes three main activities: movement to contact, which is an 880-yard run in utility pants and combat

ness, body composition, and military appearance while diminishing other risk factors in order to improve Marine combat readiness and personal appearance.

[9] Hogan, 2015, pp. 16–17.

[10] Hogan, 2015, pp. 11–16.

[11] Hogan, 2015, pp. 37.

boots; timed lifting of a 30-pound ammunition can; and maneuver under fire, which is a combination of aerobic and anaerobic activities that include carrying a fellow marine for a preset distance.[12] The addition of the CFT tracks along with the overall trend of Marine Corps fitness requirements toward elements that demand more power and strength of all marines, regardless of gender. Although the CFT and PFT both include gender- and age-normed scoring, the gaps in required performance standards between men and women have decreased over time, even as fitness standards have increased across the board.[13]

Repeal of the Direct-Ground Combat Definition and Assignment Rule

In addition to changes in the fitness tests, the Marine Corps has also revised policies that expand the role of women in the force. The result of these policies is that women are allowed to officially fill roles that are more physically demanding than those they were historically assigned to. In 2013, the Secretary of Defense repealed the Direct Ground Combat Definition and Assignment Rule, which had been in place since 1994. This effectively opened up all ground combat specialties to women, enabling them to start training and qualifying for more physically demanding roles in the Marine Corps.

With the opening of these previously closed MOSs, in addition to changes in overall fitness standards per the CFT and PFT, physical standards for specific ground combat MOSs have been developed and published. These standards require any marine, regardless of gender, assigned to these specific MOSs to achieve a higher fitness level than the PFT and CFT alone demand, with clear and detailed requirements spelled out in each Training and Readiness Manual. These new standards can lead marines to build muscle in ways that can challenge existing body-composition and height/weight standards.

---

[12] MCO 6100.13A CH-3, 2021.

[13] See Hogan, 2015; and Jeff Schogol, "The PFT and CFT Can Be Gender Neutral. Here's How," *Marine Times*, July 10, 2017.

For example, the artillery MOS, which, until repeal of the Direct Ground Combat Definition and Assignment Rule, had been closed to women, now requires artillery marines to wear and carry a fighting load (54.35 lbs.) while

1. lifting a 75.6-lb. Mk19 grenade launcher to a tactical vehicle (simulated by lifting from ground to overhead)
2. ensuring a casualty is not under direct fire (moving 50 meters while dragging a partner).

Furthermore, marines must wear the crew uniform with proper protective equipment (19.38 lbs.) while

1. placing the 95-lb. 155mm M107 projectile on an M777 loading tray (lifting it and carrying it 5 meters five separate times in 75 seconds)
2. preparing ammunition for displacement (lifting and carrying the same 95-lb. ammunition 50 meters five times in 4 minutes and 56 seconds).

And finally, marines must wear the utility uniform to perform a single lift of a simulated casualty onto the bed of a tactical vehicle, simulated by a single clean-and-press repetition of a 115-lb. weight bar.[14]

These exercises are demanding and require the development and maintenance of muscle and mass. The development of lean muscle mass can lead to weight gain and, as we explore in a later section, problematic BMI estimates.

It is important to understand the differences in standards to meet occupational requirements and the standards to meet physical fitness requirements, because these often become conflated. As has been outlined, the goal of physical fitness standards set by the PFT and CFT is to measure general functional fitness and overall health, whereas MOS-specific standards inform a marines' ability to serve in a specific combat specialty. Although changes in both MOS standards and fitness standards have

[14] Navy Marine Corps 3500.7C, *Artillery Training and Readiness Manual*, Washington, D.C.: Department of the Navy, Headquarters United States Marine Corps, October 29, 2018.

impact on the BCMAP, because their objectives are different, they should not be conflated.

Comparison of Standards to Other Services

Although DoD provides guidance for the services when it comes to BCAs, there is latitude granted to each of the services to provide for their respective requirements as long as they are not more lenient than DoD's standard. Although each service has different requirements, understanding their respective approaches places the Marine Corps policy in context. Although all four of the services conduct a body composition and PFA,[15] the U.S. Air Force is the only one exempt from the DoD standard of using body fat percentage. The Air Force instead incorporates an abdominal-circumference measurement as a component of its PFA, but, as of December 2020, it has eliminated the use of the measurement as the service further explores the need for the requirement.[16] The Air Force plans to establish a separate assessment of body composition that will start in October 2021, in accordance with DoDI 1308.3, which establishes a requirement for assessment. The Army also is reevaluating its body-composition program to determine the future of the program and to study concerns related to the tape test.[17] Table 2.3 summarizes the objective, method of measurement, and body fat percentage requirement for each of the services.

Each of the service policies differs in its specific requirements and implementation. For instance, each service has different policies to conduct height and weight assessments. The U.S. Army encourages commanders to allow seven days between weigh-ins and the PFT to ensure that weigh-ins do not interfere with a soldier's performance on the fitness test. The Navy mandates that its BCA be conducted no less than ten days but no closer than 24 hours prior to their physical readiness test. For all services, height

[15] U.S. Air Force, U.S. Army, Marine Corps, and U.S. Navy. Currently, the U.S. Space Force is still developing its body-composition policies.

[16] Pawlyk, 2020.

[17] Davis Winkie, "No More Tape Test? Army Study to Reevaluate Body Fat Program," *Army Times*, July 20, 2021.

TABLE 2.3
Comparison of Service Body Composition Standards

Service	Objective	Method of Measurement	Maximum Body Fat Percentage	Policy
DoD	Service members shall maintain physical readiness through appropriate nutrition, health, and fitness habits. Aerobic capacity, muscular strength, muscular endurance, and desirable body fat composition form the basis for the DoD physical fitness and body fat programs.	BMI table is used for height-weight screening; body fat must be calculated using circumference-based method.	DoD policy states that the services can have a stricter standard but not a more liberal or lenient standard. The services cannot have body fat percentages that exceed 36 percent for women and 26 percent for men.	DoDI 1308.3
Air Force	Motivate all airmen to participate in a year-round physical conditioning program that emphasizes total fitness, including proper aerobic conditioning, muscular fitness training, and healthy eating; increase productivity, optimize health, and decrease absenteeism while maintaining a higher level of readiness.	As of December 2020, the Air Force removed its abdominal circumference measurement. Separate BCA to begin in October 2021.	N/A	Air Force Manual 36-2905[a]

TABLE 2.3—CONTINUED

Service	Objective	Method of Measurement	Maximum Body Fat Percentage	Policy
Army	Ensure all soldiers achieve and maintain optimal well-being and performance under all conditions; establish and maintain operational readiness, physical fitness, health, and professional military appearance.	Height for weight is based on tables; circumference-based taping (men: neck and waist; women: neck, hip, and waist).	Age group: 17–20; men: 20 percent; women: 30 percent. Age group: 21–27; men: 22 percent; women: 32 percent. Age group: 28–39; men: 24 percent; women: 34 percent. Age group: 40 and older; men: 26 percent; women: 36 percent.	Army Regulation 600-9[b]
Marine Corps	Establish healthy weight and body-composition standards and ensure all marines present a suitable military appearance; contribute to the health and well-being of every marine; motivate marines to set the example.	Height for weight is based on tables; circumference-based taping (men: neck and waist; women: neck, hip, and waist).	Age group: 17–25; men: 18 percent; women: 26 percent. Age group: 26–35; men: 19 percent; women: 27 percent. Age group: 36–45; men: 20 percent; women: 28 percent. Age group: 46 and older; men: 21 percent; women: 29 percent.	MCO 6110.3A

TABLE 2.3—CONTINUED

Service	Objective	Method of Measurement	Maximum Body Fat Percentage	Policy
Navy	It is important for all Navy personnel to maintain a minimum prescribed level of physical fitness necessary for worldwide deployment, whenever or wherever needed; the Navy uses a holistic approach to overall wellness via exercise, nutrition, weight control, tobacco cessation, prevention of alcohol abuse, and health and wellness education.	There is a three-step process: (1) height for weight based on tables; (2) if not within height/weight, a single abdominal-circumference measurement; and (3) if not within abdominal-circumference limits, circumference-based taping (men: neck and waist; women: neck, hip, and waist).	Abdominal circumference: women: 35.5 in.; men: 39 in. Body fat: women: 36 percent; men: 26 percent	Office of Naval Operations Instruction 6110.1J[c]

[a] Air Force Manual 36-2905, *Air Force Physical Fitness Program*, Washington, D.C.: Secretary of the Air Force, December 11, 2020.
[b] Army Regulation 600-9, 2019.
[c] Office of Naval Operations Instruction 6110.1J, *Physical Readiness Program*, Washington, D.C.: Department of the Navy, Office of the Chief of Naval Operations, July 11, 2011.

and weight is a semiannual requirement. Administrative actions for those who fail a BCA are fairly standard across the services that conduct them (as of this writing, the Air Force does not). Administrative actions associated with a failure include being ineligible for promotion or advancement, written documentation on fitness reports and the service file, being ineligible for command, and being ineligible for assignment to special training. Once an individual passes the BCP, that service member is again eligible for those aspects of service that were previously restricted.

The services differ in their thresholds for administrative separation related to body composition. For the Army, unsatisfactory progress toward weight loss over two consecutive months or failure to meet standards after six months results in processing for administrative separation. Additionally, soldiers who fail to meet standards within 12 months of BCP completion will be separated, and those who exceed standards again within 36 months will be given 90 days to meet the standard or be separated. The Navy does not administratively separate its enlisted sailors for PFA failures (a failed body composition is considered a PFA failure). Enlisted sailors are ineligible for retention or advancement and will be separated at the end of their obligated service unless they pass a PFA and reinstate their ability to be retained. For officers, a one-time failure of the PFA results in adverse documentation, but eligibility for promotion can be regained upon passage of the next PFA. Two consecutive failures result in processing for separation at the officer's projected rotation date.

The intent of each services' body-composition policy differs, as does what each service emphasizes to be the policy's intent. According to the Defense Health Board, the Marine Corps, which has the lowest body fat percentage requirements of all the services, upholds this requirement because it has a culture that "places a high priority on appearance."[18] In the introductory section of the BCMAP, the order states,

> Marines who exceed weight and body fat standards are a detriment to and detract from the combat readiness of their unit. . . . The presentation of an unsuitable military appearance is inconsistent with the Marine Corps leadership principle of setting the example. Simply put, Marines who do not present a suitable military appearance fail to possess the qualities necessary to effectively lead Marines.[19]

The Air Force prioritizes body composition as a component of overall fitness. Recently, the Chief of Staff of the Air Force made comments about the service's decision to eliminate the abdominal circumference measurement from the PFA. "We believe these potential test structure changes will impact airmen in a positive way and help with a holistic approach to health and fitness standards," he said.[20] Recent changes to the Navy's order include a three-step method of BCA measurement and other changes aimed to better achieve the balance between health and the unique requirements of the increasingly technical nature of many Navy jobs.

Service policies also include other differences. For instance, the Navy's and Army's body-composition policies specifically prohibit personnel from

[18] Defense Health Board, 2013.

[19] MCO 6110.3A, 2019, p. 1-1.

[20] Quoted in Pawlyk, 2020.

harmful habits, such as using body wraps, starvation diets, and sauna suits, to change their body measurements. Army policy includes sections related to unsafe weight-loss strategies, diets, and eating disorders.

Conclusion

Marine Corps body-composition standards were established in the 1970s. Since then, the Marine Corps has adapted these standards incrementally to address changes in force population, adjust to changes to physical fitness requirements, and meet congressional demands. The conflict is between (1) a desire to set strict policy to address concerns about rising obesity trends and (2) a need to respond to concerns that the restrictive standards are adversely impacting specific populations. The incremental nature of the changes suggests a failure to look at the policy more holistically and determine how changes to policy will affect the force.

Marine Corps policies meet DoD requirements for BCPs and are aligned with other services' policies. Compared with the other services, the Marine Corps' body fat percentage standard is the strictest, and the service places a heavier emphasis on the need to maintain personal appearance. The physical requirements levied on a marine today require increasing muscle and mass, which is at odds with Marine Corps policy encouraging a "lean and trim" marine.

CHAPTER THREE

Scientific Basis for Body Composition Standards

As noted earlier, MCO 6110.3A aligns with DoD's policy on body composition. Adopted in 2017, the most recent changes in 2019 and 2021 aimed at establishing pregnancy and postpartum policy. Despite the updates, the order's basic inputs—height and weight tables, body fat scoring, and the taping method—are not new and reflect the populations from which they were developed. However, over the past 25 years, physical performance and fitness requirements for male and female marines have changed notably, as has the body of knowledge about health, fitness, size, performance, and measurements of each.

Evolution of Understanding of Weight, Fitness, and Health

The research behind body composition and its relationship to weight, fitness, and health is complex, and new relationships and factors to consider regularly emerge. This is a living field of research applied to living human beings who, in the case of the Marine Corps, are regularly subject to intense physical fitness standards, training, and experiences. Accordingly, developing and maintaining holistic, effective body-composition and fitness policies requires understanding the standards that current research support and how marines are affected by such standards.

When considering size, fitness, and health, health research consensus notes that although overall body fat is a general indicator of health, understanding how fat is distributed throughout the body—and not just the amount of fat—is key to assessing health. Abdominal fat—which can be estimated through waist circumference (WC) or waist-to-hip measurements—is more important than overall body fat when considering risks to health.[1] Having more visceral fat, which is located in the abdominal area and around critical organs, is positively linked to risk for cardiac disease, Type 2 diabetes, liver disease, and cancers.[2] Additionally, research supports the idea that the ratio between weight and height—or thinness—is less important to health than the body composition. Body composition measurements can determine the amount of fat carried; a healthy ratio of fat to muscle in the body is a more reliable assessment of health and fitness.[3]

Evolutions in Body Composition Measurement Methods

Along with knowledge about body composition and its relationship with fitness and health, the collective understanding of how to measure body fat, body composition, and health—and what those measurements represent—have also evolved. First, we will cover the evolution of our understanding of what height and weight and BMI measurements represent. Then we will discuss how body-composition measurements and their reliability and practicality have changed.

BMI, identified in DoDI 1308.3 as a measure of health, is used globally to track individual health and nutritional status. However, BMI has a complicated relationship with body composition. BMI without context can be misleading, because the number generated cannot separate fat and lean

[1] Magnus Borga, Janne West, Jimmy D. Bell, Nicholas C. Harvey, Thobias Romu, Steven B. Heymsfield, and Olof Dahlqvist Leinhard, "Advanced Body Composition Assessment: From Body Mass Index to Body Composition Profiling," *Journal of Investigative Medicine*, Vol. 66, No. 5, June 2018.

[2] Borga et al., 2018.

[3] Dana L. Duren, Richard J. Sherwood, Stefan A. Czerwinski, Miryoung Lee, Audrey C. Choh, Roger M. Siervogel, and Wm. Cameron Chumlea, "Body Composition Methods, Comparisons and Interpretation," *Journal of Diabetes Science and Technology*, Vol. 2, No. 6, November, 2008.

masses. BMI also does not represent the distribution of body fat throughout one's body.

Body fat distribution, not BMI, is a key part of understanding health.[4] Although the BMI formula is an easily accessed and used screening tool that can shed light on general health, the CDC emphasizes that it does not measure a person's fat; to measure fat, other methods are needed. The CDC also mentions that "athletes may have a high BMI because of increased muscularity rather than increased body fatness."[5]

Additionally, BMI was invented in the 19th century by a Belgian statistician, who developed the measure from a pool of White, European men, which could be problematic for application beyond that population.[6] Indeed, as research demonstrates, a diverse group of people can carry different amounts of body fat at the same BMI. According to the CDC, at a constant BMI, women carry more body fat than men; Asian people carry more body fat than White people, who carry more body fat than Black people; older people have more body fat than younger people; and nonathletes carry more body fat than athletes.[7]

The fact that athletes have less body fat than nonathletes at the same BMI is a critical piece of information to consider for those individuals, such as marines, who belong to populations that are required to build and maintain a higher-than-average level of physical fitness. A study performed on a group of healthy young adult women in 2018 found that, after introducing two treatment groups to two different versions of high-intensity interval training programming, both groups had lost body fat and gained muscle mass while increasing weight and BMI after 12 weeks.[8] This is an important consideration given the age and relative fitness levels of—and increased

---

[4] Jonathan C. K. Wells and M. S. Fewtrell, "Measuring Body Composition," *Archives of Disease in Childhood*, Vol. 91, No. 7, June 2006; Borga et al., 2018.

[5] Centers for Disease Control and Prevention, 2021.

[6] H. B. Kitzinger and B. Karle, *The Epidemiology of Obesity*, Vol. 45, Vienna, Austria: Springer Vienna, 2013; Carly Stern, "Why BMI Is a Flawed Health Standard, Especially for People of Color," *Washington Post*, May 5, 2021.

[7] Centers for Disease Control and Prevention, 2021.

[8] Elise C. Brown, Tamara Hew-Butler, Charles R. C. Marks, Scotty J. Butcher, and Myung D. Choi, "The Impact of Different High-Intensity Interval Training Protocols on

physical demands on—marines. Although height and weight measurements are not BMI, BMI is derived directly from height and weight, with a conversion factor.[9] This raises questions about the Marine Corps' reliance on height and weight tables to set standards. Because of this known problem with BMI as a measurement, the Marine Corps policy does not rely on BMI itself; to complement height and weight as a measure of health and fitness, the services estimate body fat.

Body composition measurement on a living human being is always an estimation, because the gold standard for measurement of body composition is cadaver analysis.[10] However, for a variety of health and fitness reasons, individual body composition needs to occasionally be measured. To answer the demand for accessible, accurate, and practical methods of assessing body composition, a series of simple to multicomponent models have emerged. Each of these methods comes with its own set of assumptions, and each introduces—often through those assumptions—one or more errors. The Marine Corps, in compliance with DoDI 1308.3, currently uses the basic, field-expedient taping method, which comes with its own assumptions and potential errors.

Current methods of body-composition measurement range from simple measurements, such as the taping method, to higher, multicomponent methods. Two-component methods estimate fat mass and fat-free mass; three-component models estimate water, body fat, and fat-free dry tissue; and multicomponent models further divide fat-free tissue into body mass/weight, total body volume, total body water, and bone-mineral content.[11] Two-component models are the simplest of the multicomponent methods and were developed using assumptions from measurements and analysis of male cadavers, introducing potential error through those assumptions.[12]

Body Composition and Physical Fitness in Healthy Young Adult Females," *BioResearch Open Access*, Vol. 7.1, 2018.

[9] The BMI formula is (weight[lb.] ÷ height[in.]^2) × 703.

[10] Wells and Fewtrell, 2006.

[11] Wells and Fewtrell, 2006.

[12] Rebecca Kuriyan, "Body Composition Techniques," *Indian Journal of Medical Research*, Vol. 148, No. 5, 2018, pp. 648–658.

Basic measurement methods can be used nearly anywhere and are relatively cheap to employ. These include such techniques as anthropometry (taping method) and skinfold measurements, with affiliated equations.[13] Anthropometry is noninvasive and includes BMI, neck and WC, and waist-to-hip ratio (WHR) measurements. WC measurements can be used to assess abdominal fat and are measured in a standing position to identify potential risk using abdominal fat levels. WHR measurements can be used to assess the distribution of fat across a person's body, with accuracy decreasing with greater fat.[14] Neck circumference was added to these measurements in recent years to potentially better estimate upper body fat and alleviate concerns that waist measurements can be affected by digesting food or breathing, although the usefulness of neck circumference measurements lacks consensus across the scientific community.[15] Skinfold measurements are used to predict body fat or body density, but they are primarily useful in the populations that the initial equations were based on and should not be used to compare across demographic groups. Accuracy can depend on factors ranging from calipers used to the skill of the person taking the measurements.[16] Skinfold measurements are more appropriate for measuring regional fatness than overall fatness. Advantages of both methods include ease of deployment and low cost.[17]

Additional relatively simple methods—compared with higher multi-component methods covered later—include bioelectrical impedance analysis (BIA), hydrodensitometry, air displacement plethysmography (ADP), and isotope dilution.

---

[13] Kuriyan, 2018.

[14] Kuriyan, 2018.

[15] María José Arias Téllez, Francisco M. Acosta, Guillermo Sanchez-Delgado, Borja Martinez-Tellez, Victoria Muñoz-Hernández, Wendy D. Martinez-Avila, Pontus Henriksson, and Jonatan R. Ruiz, "Association of Neck Circumference with Anthropometric Indicators and Body Composition Measured by DXA in Young Spanish Adults," *Nutrients*, Vol. 12, No. 2, February 2020.

[16] Kuriyan, 2018.

[17] Wells and Fewtrell, 2006.

BIA sends a low electric current through the body to measure impedance, under the principle that lean tissue is a good conductor, while body fat is not. BIA assumes that 73 percent of a body's fat-free mass is water. Hydration levels, limb length, activity, ovulation, and other factors can introduce error, however. And BIA is not currently available for field use or widespread applications through DoD.[18] Hydrodensitometry uses water displacement to distinguish fat mass and fat-free mass. Correcting for air volume in the lungs, total body fat can be estimated but distribution of that fat cannot; additionally, hydrodensitometry does not account for bone-mineral content or hydration variations between individuals, which introduces error.[19] It is also time-consuming and relatively invasive.[20]

Like hydrodensitometry, ADP uses displacement to distinguish between fat and fat-free mass but displacing air instead of water. BOD POD is the commercial name for the system that employs ADP. The same factors that affect accuracy for hydrodensitometry also introduce error here, however, because ADP similarly cannot account for variations in specific matter between individuals.[21] Additionally, the BOD POD is expensive; the process is fairly time-intensive, because it takes five to eight minutes per person; and few have access to it.[22] Finally, isotope dilution (hydrometry) estimates total body water by sending a tracer through body fluid and collecting samples. The process assumes a 73-percent level of hydration while dosing a subject to measure total water. This measurement can be used to estimate fat-free mass but is also fairly invasive.[23]

Beyond these "simpler" body-composition measurements are a variety of more-invasive and laboratory-based methods. These include various forms of magnetic resonance imaging and measurement of X-ray absorption.

Magnetic resonance imaging (more commonly known as MRI) is a best in breed of sorts for the estimation of body composition, including estimates

---

[18] Kuriyan, 2018.

[19] Borga et al., 2018.

[20] Kuriyan, 2018.

[21] Borga et al., 2018.

[22] Kuriyan, 2018.

[23] Kuriyan, 2018.

of various fat-free components, such as skeletal muscle mass and organ masses, along with bone marrow adipose tissue. Quantitative magnetic resonance, a relatively new method, estimates fat mass, lean mass, and total body water.[24]

Finally, dual-energy X-ray absorptiometry (DEXA) estimates body fat, muscle, and total body mineral mass by measuring the attenuation of X-rays with high and low energies. DEXA is fast and noninvasive, but it assumes constant hydration levels of the subject, and the estimate produced can be influenced by abdominal thickness.[25] More-advanced methods continue to develop, such as the whole-body potassium counter method, but none of these appears to be currently practical for widespread use by the military services. As of June 2021, the Marine Corps is running a yearlong body-composition study in which the service is measuring marines' body composition via traditional methods (height and weight and taping) and then comparing these methods with BIA, DEXA, and the BOD POD scan results. However, the study is not currently fielded widely because of lack of equipment access across the Corps, highlighting current challenges that all the services face to get accurate body-composition measurements.

Importantly, although body composition is considered the most accurate measurement of health and fitness, the lack of standardization, potential measurement inaccuracies, and wide variety of access considerations for the more highly regarded methods will continue to limit the military's use of body-composition measurement methods and will potentially require the services to reimagine how health and fitness are measured and scored for military personnel.[26]

---

[24] Kuriyan, 2018.

[25] Borga et al., 2018; Kuriyan, 2018.

[26] Nanna L. Meyer, Jorunn Sundgot-Borgen, Timothy G. Lohman, Timothy R. Ackland, Arthur D. Stewart, Ronald J. Maughan, Suzanne Smith, and Wolfram Müller, "Body Composition for Health and Performance: A Survey of Body Composition Assessment Practice Carried Out by the Ad Hoc Research Working Group on Body Composition, Health and Performance Under the Auspices of the IOC Medical Commission," *British Journal of Sports Medicine*, Vol. 47, No. 16, 2013.

Conclusion

In sum, because weight-to-height measurements are not direct predictors of an individual's health and fitness, other methods of assessment have developed over time. BMI is a flawed tool, originating from research using an unrepresentative sample of people, and it cannot differentiate fat from muscle mass. To better assess health and fitness, body-composition measurements have emerged over time. However, existing methods of assessing body composition, from the simplest to the most complex, come with their own assumptions and potential flaws. In the end, none of the methods we just outlined presents a clear alternative method for the services because of invasiveness, costs, and accessibility.

CHAPTER FOUR

Impacts of Body-Composition Standards on Individual Health

The body-composition and military-appearance standards codified by the BCMAP are intended to support the growth and maintenance of a fit, healthy force that can handle the rigors of combat and training in today's Marine Corps. On the surface, these standards can appear to be a sensible goal, but they may have impacts that are at odds with the policy's intended objectives. Specifically, the policy may lead to the development of negative behaviors in addition to intended positive behaviors.

In the following sections, we explore what is known about negative behaviors that can develop as a result of policies, such as the BCMAP, and in cultures that praise fitness and thinness; what is known about the prevalence of these behaviors in the Marine Corps, military, and veteran populations; and why service members are at higher risk for developing risky behaviors. We then explore potential near- and long-term impacts of these risky behaviors and how they potentially shape the long-term health of the force.

Research has identified negative behaviors as associated with health and body-composition maintenance and control in the general population; in the service member community, specifically among marines, negative behaviors are evident in the context of body-composition and fitness standards. This is concerning because, as research demonstrates, these behaviors often have long-term negative implications for the physical and mental health of those who develop them. For the individual marine, the adoption of risky behaviors can affect mental and physical health currently and in the future. The adoption of these behaviors can also limit cognitive functioning, impairing leadership and decisionmaking, resilience, endurance, and strength. For the Marine Corps as an institution, this could be concerning for the long-term health, fitness, readiness, and effectiveness of the force, as well as retention of marines from all demographic groups.

BCMAP and Associated Behaviors

The major behaviors that have been associated with body-composition measurements and relevant policy include restricted eating and/or drinking and fasting; the use of diet pills, laxatives, or diuretics; self-induced vomiting; excessive exercise; and the use of saunas and other sweat-inducing or dehydrating methods to lose weight quickly. These behaviors can affect an individual's physical and mental health, both in the short- and long-term, to say nothing of affecting decisionmaking, executive function, or physical strength and resilience in stressful situations, such as combat.[1] In the later subsection about statistics, we present known statistics about the prevalence and likely prevalence of these behaviors and the rates of diagnosis in the Marine Corps, the military in general, and veteran populations. We also cite comparable statistics, when useful, in the general civilian population.

To understand the severity of and risk inherent in these behaviors, we note that these behaviors are also the same as those identified with disordered eating; depending on the degree of behavior, the behaviors are also linked with diagnosed eating disorders per the Diagnostic and Statistical Manual of Mental Disorders (DSM-5).[2]

[1] Lindsay Bodell, Katherine Jean Forney, Pamela Keel, Peter Gutierrez, and Thomas E. Joiner, "Consequences of Making Weight: A Review of Eating Disorder Symptoms and Diagnoses in the US Military," *Clinical Psychology*, Vol. 21, No. 4, 2014; Rosemary Donalson, *Disordered Eating in Female Veterans with Military Trauma*, dissertation, San Francisco, Calif.: California Institute of Integral Studies, 2016; McNulty, 2001.

[2] "Feeding and Eating Disorders," American Psychiatric Associate, 2013.

What Are Eating Disorders and Disordered Eating?

Per the American Psychiatric Association, *eating disorders*

> are behavioral conditions characterized by severe and persistent disturbance in eating behaviors and associated distressing thoughts and emotions. They can be very serious conditions affecting physical, psychological and social function.[3]

We cover anorexia nervosa (AN), bulimia nervosa (BN), binge-eating disorder (BED), and eating disorder not otherwise specified (EDNOS) in this chapter. BEDs are at times included with BN and EDNOS.[4]

AN is shaped by an intense fear of weight or fat gain, leading patients to restrict food intake, often resulting in low body weight. AN rates are higher among younger women, the disease has subtypes that include both persistent calorie restriction and binge-and-restrict behavior, and those with AN often cross over to BN at some point. AN is one of the most serious disorders because of the physical and psychological comorbidities it carries—from depression and suicide to significant bone mass loss and body system shutdown.[5] BN, often diagnosed at higher rates than AN and generally present more broadly among women of all ages, manifests through binge-eating episodes, surrounded by a feeling of loss of control, followed by episodes of compensatory behavior, such as "vomiting, laxatives, fasting, or excessive exercise."[6] BN is easily hidden by those suffering from it. BN has two main subtypes: the purging type and the non-purging type. The purging type manifests through binge eating and related behaviors, such as vomiting, laxative, or diuretic abuse, while the non-purging type tends to manifest through fasting or excessive exercise. Despite the differences,

---

[3] American Psychiatric Association, "What Are Eating Disorders?" webpage, March 2021.

[4] Leslie A. Sim, Donald E. McAlpine, Karen B. Grothe, Susan M. Himes, Richard G. Cockerill, and Matthew M. Clark, "Identification and Treatment of Eating Disorders in the Primary Care Setting," *Mayo Clinic Proceedings*, Vol. 85, No. 8, August 2010.

[5] Sim et al., 2010.

[6] Donalson, 2016, p. 19.

the physical and mental comorbidities can be similar to those with AN. Although BN is harder to diagnose through a physical exam because the associated behaviors are more easily hidden than for AN, higher BN diagnosis rates suggest that its underlying prevalence compared with AN is even greater than rates suggest.[7]

BED manifests through "the consumption of large amounts of food in a 2-hour time period, accompanied by a perceived loss of control," repeated regularly and often followed by feelings of depression or disgust.[8] The difference between BED and BN is the lack of compensatory behavior after the binge-eating episode. BED behavior also can be hidden, although it can be accompanied by weight gain. It is more prevalent among those who are overweight or obese and can lead to comorbidities more common with weight-control issues.[9] EDNOS behavior is characterized by many of the behaviors just described but that "fall outside the specified diagnostic criteria of AN or BN."[10] This can mean anything from disordered behavior that comes in cycles to BED or AN behavior that does not hit every diagnostic criterion.

Disordered eating behavior replicates these symptoms, but the behavior may not reach the levels of frequency or duration required for a full diagnosis. Despite this, individuals demonstrating disordered eating behavior may still suffer in ways similar to those who have been formally diagnosed and may demonstrate higher levels of disordered eating behavior at particularly stressful or challenging times, such as during fitness or height/weight testing windows.[11] These individuals can still suffer short- and long-term mental and physical impacts from their behavior just as those with full eating disorders can.

---

[7] Sim et al., 2010, p. 748.

[8] Sim et al., 2010, p. 748.

[9] Sim et al., 2010, p. 749.

[10] Sim et al., 2010, p. 750.

[11] Donalson, 2016, p. 19.

Statistics for Disordered Eating and Eating Disorder Diagnoses in DoD

We can draw several observations about these behaviors and their impacts on individuals and institutions from existing research on eating disorders and on disordered eating behavior and from information about their manifestation and prevalence within military, veteran, and civilian populations.

Research about individual marine behavior in response to the Marine Corps' body-composition policy and diagnosis rates for eating disorders is sparse, as is research into similar trends across the services and in the veteran population. Here, we present a brief discussion that draws some comparisons of related behaviors in the broader civilian population, where research is developed enough to build a sense of the possible impacts of the Marine Corps' policy. We identify where specific statistics uniquely reflect relevant marine populations, service members and veterans more generally, or people writ large. Some of these behaviors are persistent, recurring regularly and consistently throughout a marine's life, while some increase and decrease with annual fitness cycles. Notably, marine behavior represented by some of the statistics captured appears to be more extreme than behavior across the other services.[12]

It is also important to recognize that, because studies of disordered eating behavior patterns and impacts in the military have been relatively rare compared with research of civilian populations, the impacts of body-composition policies, measurement methods, expectations, and career implications for service members are less understood and cataloged. As a result, pointing to eating disorder diagnosis rates alone across the services may significantly underestimate the prevalence of behavior. Although diagnoses are rare, eating disorders are among the most common and most easily hidden mental health conditions, and the military lifestyle and culture is primed to hide risky behavior.[13] Additionally, a service member can be

---

[12] See Patricia Kime, "Congress Wants the Pentagon to Expand Coverage for Troops' Eating Disorder Treatments," *Military.com*, August 12, 2020, and McNulty, 2001, for examples.

[13] Kime, 2020.

separated from the service for an eating disorder diagnosis if the illness does not respond to treatment or interrupts the performance of duties.[14] Given the persistent behavior that we outline in this chapter, the risks for service members associated with disclosing disordered eating behavior are likely very real. The stigma associated with eating disorders, along with the expectation that they mainly affect women, potentially serves to shift attention from the phenomenon or mask its existence among service members.[15]

As noted earlier, looking primarily at those who are assigned to weight control groups or who are separated from the service for failing to meet height and weight standards will miss a potentially larger population of marines—and all service members—who are at risk of failing to meet standards and therefore may exhibit behaviors relating to eating disorders. This population includes those who undertake concerning or harmful behaviors to meet standards and avoid personal or career implications.[16] As a result, it is important to study the behavior patterns associated with body composition and explore the possible long-term implications of such behaviors—beyond simply looking at diagnosis rates and survey data—to develop a more comprehensive understanding of potential impacts of body-composition policies and areas to focus further research.

According to recent diagnosis rates collected by DoD, eating disorder diagnoses rates are relatively low across the services. The diagnosis data that exist suggest that military women between 20 and 24 years old are at highest risk of developing eating disorders. Marines have been diagnosed with eating disorders at nearly twice the rate of other services, and female marines in particular have the highest rate of diagnosis across the services and all groups. Female service members stand out in general across the services as well: The diagnosis rate among female service members from

[14] Silas, 2020.

[15] Brooke A. Bartlett and Karen S. Mitchell, "Eating Disorders and Military and Veteran Men and Women: A Systematic Review," *International Journal of Eating Disorders*, Vol. 48, No. 8, December 2015; Bodell et al., 2014, pp. 398–399.

[16] Bartlett and Mitchell, 2015; Bodell et al., 2014; and Silas, 2020.

2013 to 2017 was 11 times that of their peers who are men.[17] Table 4.1 shows diagnosis rates from 2013 to 2017.

However, as just stated, the problem is suspected to be much more prevalent than diagnosis rates show. Research suggests that the prevalence of disordered eating behavior among service members is higher than the rates show and higher than in the general population, and that women are disproportionately affected.[18]

Academic research observations, particularly those that use sampling or survey data instead of diagnosis rates, reflect these numbers. When service members are asked to report their behavior without fear of repercussion, reports of risky behaviors associated with eating disorders are disturbingly high. Analyses of samples of active-duty women and female West Point cadets in the late 1990s and early 2000s found that approximately 20–29.6 percent of female cadets and 33.6 percent of active-duty Army women were at high risk of having an eating disorder—compared with approximately 10–16 percent of college women sampled in different studies.[19] A 2001 analysis of a large sample of active-duty female service members across the services—more than 3,600 service women—for both routine and episodic disordered eating behaviors found that 1.1 percent of women in the sample demonstrated symptoms of AN, 8.1 percent reported symptoms of BN, and 62.8 percent

TABLE 4.1

Comparison of Service Eating Disorder Diagnosis Rates, 2013–2017

Service	Diagnosis Rate (Men)	Diagnosis Rate (Women)
Army	1.2	11.9
Navy	0.8	11.4
Air Force	0.9	10.4
Marine Corps	1.1	20.4

SOURCE: Armed Forces Health Surveillance Branch, published in Kime, 2020.
NOTE: Rates are per 10,000 members.

[17] Kime, 2020.

[18] For examples of supporting research, see Bartlett and Mitchell, 2015; and Bodell et al., 2014.

[19] Bodell et al., 2014, p. 400.

of the sample demonstrated symptoms of EDNOS.[20] Notably, the marines who were surveyed—the entire population of female marines on Okinawa at the time—demonstrated higher rates of these disorders. Of the marines surveyed, 4.9 percent of women reported symptoms of AN, 15.9 percent of BN, and a 76.7 percent of EDNOS.[21] Reported behavior included both routine and episodic use of laxatives, diuretics, and diet pills and vomiting, fasting, and excessive exercise. Table 4.2 presents the disordered eating behavior rates, both routine or episodic, identified in this 2001 analysis.

Additionally, although some of these behaviors might not be frequent or consistent enough to reach the full eating disorder diagnosis threshold, research demonstrates that situational disordered eating behavior, such as the kind developed around the timing of fitness and related height/weight testing, can be severe in the services. A set of interviews among active-duty women conducted in 1999 found that 39 percent of respondents displayed situational disorder eating behaviors as fitness testing windows approached.[22]

Specific to the Marine Corps, the 2001 survey just described found that year-round routine employment of risky behaviors occurred for women across the services but that these behaviors were also episodic, peaking

TABLE 4.2
Estimated Disordered Eating Rates, 2001

Service	AN Behavior	BN Behavior	EDNOS Behavior
Army	1.3%	4.3%	57.4%
Navy	1.1%	5.2%	61.2%
Air Force	0.8%	9.3%	58.6%
Marines	4.9%	15.9%	76.7%

SOURCE: McNulty, 2001, pp. 54–55.
NOTES: *N* = 1,278 active-duty women: Army (*n* =235), Navy (*n* = 443), Air Force (*n* = 355), Marine Corps (*n* = 245).

[20] McNulty, 2001, p. 53.

[21] McNulty, 2001, p. 53.

[22] Seibert, 2007.

around fitness and weight testing. Both routine and episodic employment of disordered eating behaviors also occurred at a higher rate among marines.[23] Additionally, compared with other service women, female marines were significantly more likely to be of below-average weight,[24] which is an area for further study to understand why this occurs.

Table 4.3 captures the 2001 sample analysis of routine behaviors cataloged by service women.

Additionally, disordered eating behaviors reported at episodic peak times included the use of diet pills (29 percent reported daily use in conjunction with fitness testing, 19 percent reported more than daily use), laxatives (12.6 percent daily near fitness testing, 5.3 percent more than daily), diuretics (24 percent daily, 11.4 percent more than daily), vomiting (19.4 percent three to six times per week, 3 percent daily), fasting (40.6 percent during fitness testing), and excessive exercise (episodic peak use not reported in the study).

Female marines demonstrated all behaviors at higher rates than women in the other services. For example, 13.1 percent female marines reported routinely exercising twice per day, and 1.2 percent reported routinely exercising more than twice per day; in comparison, 3.9 percent Navy women reported excessively exercising.[25]

Overall, the 2001 survey found that 1.1 percent of women surveyed reported AN behavior, 8.1 percent reported BN behavior, and 62.8 percent

TABLE 4.3

Estimated Disordered Eating Behaviors (Routine Use): 2001 Sample of Active-Duty Women

Service	Water Pills	Vomiting	Fasting	Diet Pills	Laxatives	Exercise
Army	1.3%	2.6%	18.8%	8.6%	2.2%	3.4%
Navy	4.4%	2.3%	18.3%	11.2%	2.3%	3.9%
Air Force	2.9%	3.2%	20.2%	13.4%	3.4%	2.3%
Marines	6.3%	3.3%	38%	28.6%	12.4%	13.1%

SOURCE: McNulty, 2001, p. 56.

[23] McNulty, 2001, p. 53.

[24] McNulty, 2001, p. 55.

[25] McNulty, 2001, p. 56.

reported behavior aligned with EDNOS. This analysis has not been repeated or supplemented since 2001, and its findings should be interpreted with caution because of low response rates and the use of self-reported behavior. However, the stigma or career implications associated with reporting disordered eating behavior necessitates employment of a variety of research methods, including gathering survey data, to better assess the problem. Similar behavior patterns have been observed among military men as well—suggesting that prevalence is also higher among these service members than among civilian men. A 2005 self-reported survey of active-duty Navy men and women found that 15 percent of respondents reported overexercising, 25 percent regularly fasted, approximately one-third reported binge-type behaviors, 5 percent used vomiting to purge, and 18 percent used laxatives.[26] An analysis of nearly 3,000 service members via anonymous survey two decades ago found that nearly 23 percent of respondents, military men and women alike, reported using some kind of unhealthy weight-control behavior to comply with body-composition requirements. These behaviors were reported in 31.2 percent of women and 20.54 percent of men; male marines in particular were more likely to engage in these behaviors than members of the other services.

And although female service members were 2.9 times more likely to demonstrate these behaviors than their male counterparts in the 2001 analysis, other studies found the opposite.[27] A 1997 analysis of Navy men and disordered eating found a higher prevalence of concerning behavior than among Navy women, suggesting that although the two genders experience the problem differently, men are still at high risk.[28] A survey of primarily enlisted White men in the Navy over the same period found that nearly 23 percent of respondents reported using a variety of disordered eating behavior to comply with existing body-composition standards. Respondents reported using laxatives, diuretics, diet pills, and self-induced vomiting to lose weight.[29]

[26] Bartlett and Mitchell, 2015, p. 1060.

[27] Seibert, 2007, pp. 47–48.

[28] Seibert, 2007, p. 17.

[29] Seibert, 2007, p. iii.

Unfortunately, as of this writing, no published research has examined potential demographic group differences beyond gender in the development and reinforcement of eating disorder behaviors among marines or any service members. This is a notable gap in the literature and of particular concern, given the potentially disproportionate impacts that the BCMAP may have on people of color, particularly women of color, and the behaviors just described.

Research about disordered eating among veterans, scarce as it is, displays similar trends of disordered eating behavior, demonstrating how long such behaviors can continue to affect individuals' lives. Phone interviews with female veterans in 2012 found that 15.6 percent reported eating disorder symptoms during their lifetimes.[30] Analysis of the prevalence of mental health issues of Iraq and Afghanistan veterans found that women reported higher rates of disordered eating behaviors than men—and that these behaviors were more likely to be associated with higher posttraumatic stress disorder (PTSD), depression, and alcohol abuse.[31] Additionally, these behaviors were associated with physical issues, such as weight gain and obesity, which are identified problems in the veteran population. In fact, health care costs associated with obesity are already high, particularly for the U.S. Department of Veterans Affairs (VA), which estimates that it spends approximately $1.67 billion annually for diabetes alone within the veteran population.[32]

Despite observable impacts across genders, female veterans as a whole again seem disproportionately affected. They had lower BMIs and significantly higher rates of eating because of emotional and stressful reasons than their male peers. They reported more binge eating, loss of control feelings, and purging behavior.[33] Other trends emerge from the research: A

[30] Bodell et al., 2014, p. 402.

[31] Jennifer D. Slane, Michele D. Levine, Sonya Borrero, Kristin M. Mattocks, Amy D. Ozler, Norman Silliker, Harini Bathulapalli, Cynthia Brandt, and Sally G. Haskell, "Eating Behaviors: Prevalence, Psychiatric Comorbidity, and Associations with Body Mass Index Among Male and Female Iraq and Afghanistan Veterans," *Military Medicine*, Vol. 181, Nos. 11–12, November–December 2016, p. 1650.

[32] Slane et al., 2016, p. 1651.

[33] Slane et al., 2016, p. 1652.

study of female veterans undertaken from 2008 to 2013 found that women who reported military sexual trauma (MST) were more than twice as likely to score as suffering from an eating disorder, women who reported sexual harassment were nearly twice as likely to have an eating disorder, and sexual harassment and rape were both significant predictors of eating disorders via multiple assessment methods.[34] Because women are already at increased risk of disordered eating because of MST, potential impacts of the BCMAP may be piling on even greater risk for women.

As noted earlier, PTSD remains strongly associated with disordered eating for female and male veterans alike. The 2008–2013 study found that female veterans with PTSD were nearly five times as likely to report AN behavior, three times more likely to report BN behavior, and more than three times more likely to report BED.[35] And veterans of all genders with disordered eating behaviors reported higher rates of depression and PTSD than their peers.[36]

Again, however, as of this writing, we could identify no significant research about the impacts on different demographic groups within the broader veteran population. This also represents a problematic gap in the literature. We strongly encourage future research to address this gap and to more accurately capture potential impacts to the short- and long-term mental and physical health of all marines, service members, and veterans alike. Given the potentially disproportionate impacts of the BCMAP on different demographic groups, it is critical to have research that assesses the BCMAP's effects on behavior of these groups to understand if inequitable policy implications are at work.

[34] Donalson, 2016, pp. 57–58.

[35] Donalson et al., 2016, p. 59.

[36] Slane et al., 2016, p. 1655.

Why Is the Military at Greater Risk for Disordered Eating Behaviors?

Although statistics vary and are more robustly captured in the civilian population, surveys of disordered eating behavior and research cataloging eating disorder symptoms among military members identify areas of concern, demonstrating that, among service members, these issues should be more thoroughly studied and addressed. Research suggests that the increased relevance of weight and body-composition measurements, the way these standards are tied to career progression and self-image, and the immersion in a culture that embraces peak fitness and appearance all combine to place service members at high risk of developing disordered eating behavior. Individuals subject to greater emphasis on shape and weight are at increased risk of developing an eating disorder in the civilian population, and the military's fitness culture and focus on body shape and weight raises warning flags.[37] But the risks for service members go far beyond these straightforward factors.

Five main themes in the military lifestyle emerge in regard to eating and military service, which can identify where military members are at greater risk. First, military service can significantly affect a service member's ability to eat and find healthful options, particularly when they are deployed to remote or hazardous environments. The homogeneity of provided food (such as meals, ready-to-eat, or MREs) and the limited selections available can also shape service members' eating behaviors and habits. Second, by linking career progression and esteem to physical measurements, military service codifies the idea that appearance and shape can determine personal value. Recall from the introduction that the BCMAP order states that

> Marines who exceed weight and body fat standards are a detriment to and detract from the combat readiness of their unit. . . . The presentation of an unsuitable military appearance is inconsistent with the Marine Corps leadership principle of setting the example. Simply

[37] Bartlett and Mitchell, 2015, p. 1065; Bodell et al., 2014.

> put, Marines who do not present a suitable military appearance fail to possess the qualities necessary to effectively lead Marines.[38]

Third, and of significant relevance for service members compared with civilians, exposure to trauma can increase the risk of developing an eating disorder in the general population, a trend that appears in military-focused research as well.[39] Service members are at increased risk of trauma from the moment they join the service and begin training. From dangerous and intense training to the preparation for and actual experience of combat, the potential for trauma can be higher in military service than in the general population. Indeed, PTSD is widely documented among veterans, with anywhere between 13 percent and 30 percent of veterans experiencing PTSD during their lifetimes.[40] Overall higher levels of insecurity, which service members are subject to through their daily work, are also linked to trauma and eating disorders.[41]

Fourth, adverse childhood experiences and adverse life experiences specifically have significant and positive links to eating disorders. Beyond combat trauma, military members report higher adverse childhood experiences scores than their civilian counterparts, experience combat trauma, and, as covered regularly in the media today, MST. These experiences are deeply linked to eating disorders of all kinds in the general population: Men who have experienced adverse experiences are more likely to be obese, while women are more likely to experience eating disorders.[42] This is particularly concerning when considering female service members because of the elevated risk of MST they face.[43] Indeed,

---

[38] MCO 6110.3A CH-1 and Admin CH, 2019, p. 1-1.

[39] Bodell et al 2014, p. 399.

[40] Miriam Reisman, "PTSD Treatment for Veterans: What's Working, What's New, and What's Next," *Pharmacy and Therapeutics*, Vol. 41, No. 10, October 2016.

[41] Seibert, 2007.

[42] Erin L. Cobb, Angela L. Lamson, Coral Steffey, Alexander M. Schoemann, and Katherine W. Didericksen, "Disordered Eating and Military Populations: Understanding the Role of Adverse Childhood Experiences," *Journal of Military, Veteran, and Family Health*, Vol. 6, No. 1, May 2020.

[43] Donalson, 2016, pp. 1–2.

a 2009 analysis found that, among female veterans seeking treatment for MST, 30–40 percent reported employing some form of disordered eating behavior.[44]

Finally, individuals at risk may also self-select into the military, because the military culture and lifestyle offers a way to hide risky behaviors while making oneself seem invulnerable.[45] A survey of female Marine Corps recruits found that 77 percent demonstrated disordered eating behavior before enlisting, 35 percent reported limiting their caloric intake, and almost 70 percent used pills or vomiting to counter bingeing behavior. Preexisting behaviors might lead predisposed individuals to the military, while military culture can reinforce or exacerbate such behaviors.[46]

These statistics and the identified increased risks that come with military service require additional research and analysis. As stated earlier, research is sparse, and many of the statistics identified in this report so far come from older studies. The potential long-term physical and mental health impacts of disordered eating offer more areas for deeper analysis. Additionally, although existing research does not explore this question in any substantive ways, women are a minority in the services, especially the Marine Corps. As a result, women in general, particularly those who come from underrepresented racial or ethnic demographic groups, can be subject to unseen and relatively understudied pressure to perform, internalize problematic experiences, or strive to overperform. These factors could place these women at even greater risk of developing eating disorder behavior. We recommend that future research efforts include an exploration of cultural and demographic considerations to capture the potential impacts of the BCMAP policy and related behavior on diverse service members.[47]

---

[44] Donalson, 2016, p. 2.

[45] Bodell et al., 2014, pp. 398–399.

[46] Bartlett and Mitchell, 2015.

[47] Emerald A. Archer, "The Power of Gendered Stereotypes in the U.S. Marine Corps," *Armed Forces and Society*, Vol. 39, No. 2, 2013.

CHAPTER FIVE

Impacts of Body-Composition Standards on Long-Term Health

Although rates of eating disorder diagnoses are low in the military community, the prevalence is likely much higher than recognized. Long-term physical and mental health impacts of these behaviors could have a burden on individuals and institutions. In the context of the Marine Corps, these burdens may be carried by Marine veterans, the VA, and their communities—but they may also be borne by still-serving marines and the Corps itself. Research about the potential impacts on the mental and physical health of individual marines, along with how disordered eating may affect marines' decisionmaking skills, resilience, and strength—particularly in stressful situations—is virtually nonexistent. Research about how diverse groups of marines may also be affected is similarly scarce but is equally needed. Developing this research can help the Corps identify what these impacts may be, whether they are inequitably distributed, and how they may shape the health of the force and retention. This chapter explores what is known about the possible impacts of disordered eating on the general and veteran populations, with potential implications for service members.

Long-Term Mental and Physical Health Impacts of Disordered Eating

A longitudinal study of middle-age civilian women and disordered eating found that nearly 11 percent of the survey group reported disordered eating behavior. Among the respondents, those exhibiting disordered eating demonstrated "significantly poorer mental and physical quality of life," sustained over time.[1] Indeed, the significant differences in quality of life between those exhibiting disordered eating behaviors and those who did not was sustained over time and greater than the differences associated with major illnesses, such as cancer.[2] These findings echo other longitudinal analyses that similarly identified links among disordered eating, mental and physical health, and quality of life.

Although physical and mental health issues are often deeply linked, as they appear to be in the longitudinal study just cited, for the purposes of exploring the various possible impacts of disordered eating, we artificially bifurcate them in the following discussion.

Mental health remains a sensitive subject in the military. Service members are often reluctant to disclose information about behaviors associated with mental health because of the stigma of mental health disorders in the military. This is compounded by the stigma that eating disorders often carry, particularly within the military.[3] Research about connections between mental health and disordered eating in the military exists, but research about these links in the veteran and civilian populations is more robust. Analyses of long-term consequences for individuals demonstrating disordered eating behavior in these populations identified links between disordered eating behaviors and mental health years later and found that disordered eating is associated with depression, anxiety, obsessive-compulsive disorder, PTSD, and, as referenced, lower-rated mental health quality of life. Overall depressed levels of self-confidence, combined with recurrent feelings of disgust, guilt, shame, and lifelong body issues, are also associated with eating disorders.[4]

---

[1] A. Kate Fairweather-Schmidt, Christina Lee, and Tracey D. Wade, "A Longitudinal Study of Midage Women with Indicators of Disordered Eating," *Developmental Psychology*, Vol. 51, No. 5, 2015, p. 722.

[2] Fairweather-Schmidt, Lee, and Wade, 2015, p. 727.

[3] Bodell et al., 2014, p. 399.

[4] Nancy D. Berkman, Kathleen N. Lohr, and Cynthia M. Bulik, "Outcomes of Eating Disorders: A Systematic Review of the Literature," *International Journal of Eating Disorders*, Vol. 40, No. 4, May 2007; Ulla Kärkkäinen, Linda Mustelin, Anu Raevuori, Jaakko Kaprio, and Anna Keski-Rahkonen, "Do Disordered Eating Behaviours Have Long-Term Health-Related Consequences?" *European Eating Disorders Review*, Vol. 26, No. 1, January 2018.

PTSD and depression in particular seem to be heavily associated with disordered eating among civilians and veterans alike. Individuals who report disordered eating behavior are more likely to report being depressed.[5] Similar observations in the veteran population further refine the connections among PTSD, depression, and disordered eating behaviors. According to a study on the prevalence of eating disorders among female veterans, 10 percent of those diagnosed with AN and 14.1 percent of those diagnosed with BN also had PTSD.[6] General weight problems are also associated with PTSD: In one analysis of military members performed by the Millennium Cohort Study, a positive PTSD screening result was associated with at least a ten-pound weight gain at a later follow-up.[7]

Additionally, as stated earlier, combat trauma and MST are associated with disordered eating; like in the civilian population, individuals with an eating disorder over their lifetime are far more likely to have experienced some form of trauma.[8] The "escape theory" of disordered eating suggests that these risky behaviors "function as a maladaptive coping mechanism for negative self-cognitions and affective distress" experienced by individuals, particularly for female veterans, who suffer higher rates of sexual trauma because of their experiences in the service.[9] Indeed, female veterans with

---

[5] Katie M. O'Brien, Denis R. Whelan, Dale P. Sandler, Janet E. Hall, and Clarice R. Weinberg, "Predictors and Long-Term Health Outcomes of Eating Disorders," *PLOS One*, Vol. 12, No. 7, July 2017, p. 6.

[6] Valerie L. Forman-Hoffman, Michelle Mengeling, Brenda M. Booth, James Torner, and Anne G. Sadler, "Eating Disorders, Post-Traumatic Stress, and Sexual Trauma in Women Veterans," *Military Medicine*, Vol. 177, No. 10, October 2012, pp. 1161–1163.

[7] Jennifer L. Bakalar, Marissa Barmine, Lindsay Druskin, Cara H. Olsen, Jeffrey Quinlan, Tracy Sbrocco, Marian Tanofsky-Kraff, "Childhood Adverse Life Events, Disordered Eating, and Body Mass Index in U.S. Military Service Members," *International Journal of Eating Disorders*, Vol. 51, No. 5, May 2018.

[8] Forman-Hoffman et al., 2012.

[9] J. C. Huston, A. R. Grillo, K. M. Iverson, K. S. Mitchell, and VA Boston Healthcare System, "Associations Between Disordered Eating and Intimate Partner Violence Mediated by Depression and Posttraumatic Stress Disorder Symptoms in a Female Veteran Sample," *General Hospital Psychiatry*, Vol. 58, May–June 2019, p. 80.

a history of MST registered higher eating disorder scores, which echoes research about links between trauma and disordered eating.[10]

Furthermore, feelings of disgust, guilt, and shame are significantly associated with disordered eating behavior and trauma alike. These feelings seem particularly relevant when considering the Marine Corps' and Army's body-composition and weight-control programs and policies. We discussed the verbiage in the BCMAP linking leadership, discipline, and character to height/weight standards, and it remains relevant here. Additionally, although more-recent versions of the Army Weight Control Program have removed some of these phrases, the 2006 update stated that "excessive body fat . . . connotes a lack of personal discipline," "detracts from military appearance," and "may indicate a poor state of health, physical fitness, or stamina."[11]

Although most of the research available on the mental health impacts of disordered eating focuses on veterans and civilians, the implications for the cognitive functioning and long-term mental resilience of marines—and all service members at risk of disordered eating behavior—seem significant. However, mental health impacts form only part of the picture.

Physical health impacts of disordered eating behaviors also include a wide variety of complications—issues that are also frequently associated with one another and with other physical health concerns. These impacts include low body weight or obesity, substance-abuse problems, infertility or amenorrhea, pregnancy complications, osteoporosis and osteoarthritis, and gastrointestinal problems.[12] Amenorrhea is the loss of three or more menstrual cycles, and it is associated with reproductive health problems, bone loss, and cardiac complications.[13] Substance-abuse links primarily include a greater likelihood of smoking, because cigarette smoking acts as

[10] Huston et al., 2019, p. 80.

[11] Army Regulation 600-9, 2006, p. 1.

[12] O'Brien, 2017 p. 6.

[13] Chrisandra L. Shufelt, Tina Torbati, and Erika Dutra, "Hypothalamic Amenorrhea and the Long-Term Health Consequences," *Seminars in Reproductive Medicine*, Vol. 35, No. 3, May 2017.

an appetite suppressant (whereas alcohol consumption means unwanted calories).[14]

Additional physical health associations include endocrine and metabolic disorders, cardiovascular issues, skin problems, and various issues associated with poor nutrition, dehydration, and vitamin deficiencies.[15] Furthermore, the over- and under-nutrition that can result from maintaining eating disorders can also perpetuate the cycle on their own, independently leading to obesity, anemia, diabetes, and other problems that then feed into mental health problems, such as depression and anxiety.[16] Finally, a higher mortality rate, including greater risk of suicide, was observed via longitudinal studies of those with eating disorders.[17]

Many of these physical health complications fit into the female athlete triad. Given the high levels of fitness that female service members, and marines in particular, must demonstrate, the female athlete triad poses a significant risk. The *triad* refers to the simultaneous occurrence among female athletes of menstrual dysfunction, low energy levels (as a result of disordered eating), and decreased bone-mineral density (premature osteoporosis).[18] It is a serious condition that requires interdisciplinary treatment from a team of medical professionals.[19]

The triad is a vicious circle. Female athletes often use weight loss to improve athletic training in certain sports. However, on the extreme end of the spectrum, female athletes can experience serious eating disorders such as AN and BN. The combination of intense exercise and poor nutrition or restricted caloric intake lower the amount of estrogen in the female body necessary to produce a healthy menstrual cycle. Low hormone levels lead to amenorrhea, which is the condition of one or more missed menstrual cycles.

---

[14] O'Brien, 2017, p. 8.

[15] Himmerich et al., 2021.

[16] Himmerich et al., 2021, p. 3.

[17] Berkman, Lohr, and Bulik, 2007.

[18] Taraneh Gharib Nazem, Kathryn E. Ackerman, "The Female Athlete Triad," *Sports Health*, Vol. 4, No. 4, July 2012.

[19] OrthoInfo, "Female Athlete Triad: Problems Caused by Extreme Exercise and Dieting," webpage, August 2020.

Low estrogen levels combined with poor nutrition and increased physical performance lead to bone density loss. Female athletes with premature osteoporosis are prone to stress fractures and other injuries.

First coined by the American College of Sports Medicine in 1992, the female athlete triad is most prevalent in young female athletes who participate in sports where weight loss can improve performance, appearance, outcome, or a combination of these.[20] For example, running is a sport that prioritizes thinner bodies to maximize performance. Very optical sports, such as ballet and gymnastics, value lower body weight for appearance purposes (and in some cases, to maximize performance). Rowing and martial arts are two examples of sports that classify athletes by certain body weight, thereby using weight as a measure of outcome.[21] In all three cases, a female athlete who wants to use her weight to her advantage in the sport may overtrain, coupling this with some type of disordered eating (AN, binge eating, crash diets), thus resulting in the female athlete triad.

Female Athlete Triad and the Military

It is important to differentiate measures of performance versus outcome in the case of body composition in military services. All military fitness tests are performance driven: Better performance leads to a higher score. However, the height and weight standards in the services are outcome driven: Service members "pass" as long as they are under the threshold of their maximum weight for their height, age, and gender. These metrics can be contradictory, especially for female service members who have stricter height/weight standards. Physical tests across all services have a combination of aerobic (running) and muscle-performance activities (sit-ups, push-ups, pull-ups). In the case of the new Army Combat Fitness Test (AFCT), test events emphasize muscle-building activities, such as deadlift, spring-drag-carry, and power throw.[22] As a result, soldiers—specifically

[20] Nazem and Ackerman, 2012.

[21] TeensHealth for Neumours, "Female Athlete Triad," webpage, July 2020.

[22] Haley Britzky, "How the Army Combat Fitness Test Exposes the Military's Unhealthy Focus on 'Making Weight,'" *Task and Purpose*, March 9, 2011.

women—pass the ACFT but do not pass the height/weight standards because of increased size in muscle mass from training toward the ACFT.[23] In fact, a study found that female soldiers who have a higher BMI outperform their "smaller" female counterparts in a variety of combat-related events.[24]

This disconnect between increased physical fitness performance at the cost of height/weight failure outcomes in the military can encourage women to succumb to the female athlete triad. As female service members are expected to increase physical performance, they are also simultaneously expected to maintain a certain weight that often has no indication on performance. Failing to uphold one or the other results in personnel action. The prevalence of female athlete triad among active-duty military women has not been well studied. In a 1999 study on women's health in the Army, a sample of 423 active-duty female soldiers were asked to complete an eating disorder inventory questionnaire, a gynecological interview and examination, and an X-ray to assess bone density. The doctors concluded that the full female athlete triad was not present in the sample population and that the female athlete triad is not "a clinically significant problem for the Army."[25] However, dietary restriction of the severity associated with AN would be expected to be underreported by military women and usually through informal outlets, such as social media (see Figure 5.1).[26]

Although there are few studies that explicitly link the female athlete triad in military women, several studies address the individual aspects of the triad outside the military population.

Considering the entirety of potential mental and physical health impacts associated with disordered eating on individuals, it is important to also consider how individual function can be shaped by disordered eating.

---

[23] Britzky, 2011.

[24] Wyatt Olson, "Heavier Female Soldiers Out-Perform Leaner Counterparts in Strength Tasks, Study Finds," *Military.com*, March 4, 2020.

[25] Tamara D. Lauder, Marc V. Williams, Carol S. Campbell, Gary Davis, Richard Sherman, and Elizabeth Pulos, "The Female Athlete Triad: Prevalence in Military Women," *Military Medicine*, Vol. 164, No. 9, September 1999.

[26] Institute of Medicine, 1998.

FIGURE 5.1

Thread from a Public Facebook Post About a Female Marine's Efforts to Meet Height and Weight Standards in June 2021

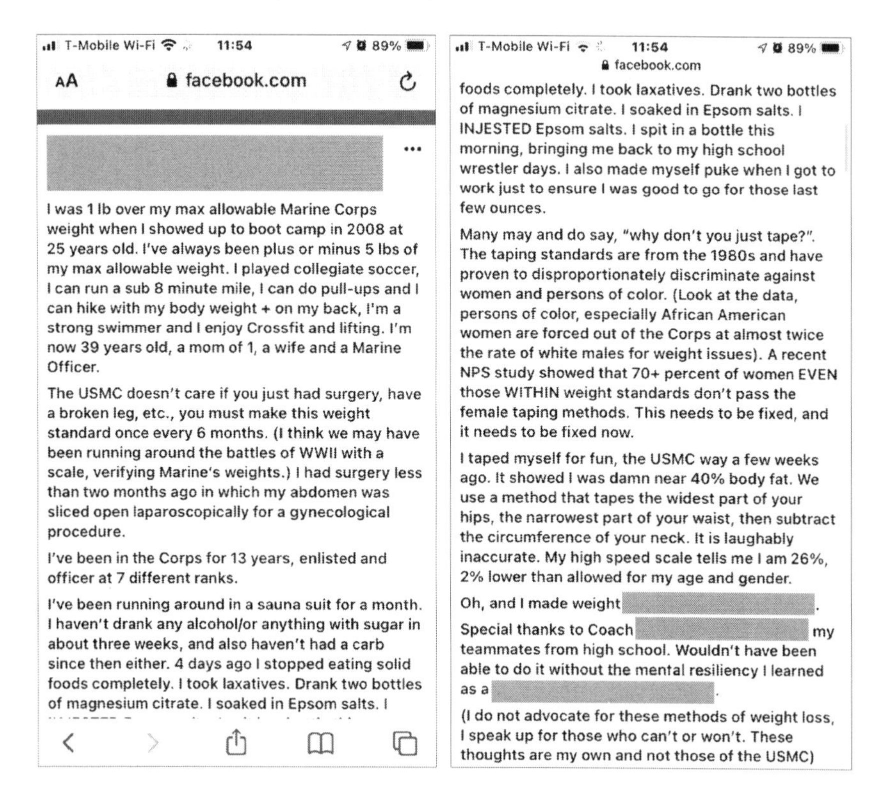

I was 1 lb over my max allowable Marine Corps weight when I showed up to boot camp in 2008 at 25 years old. I've always been plus or minus 5 lbs of my max allowable weight. I played collegiate soccer, I can run a sub 8 minute mile, I can do pull-ups and I can hike with my body weight + on my back, I'm a strong swimmer and I enjoy Crossfit and lifting. I'm now 39 years old, a mom of 1, a wife and a Marine Officer.

The USMC doesn't care if you just had surgery, have a broken leg, etc., you must make this weight standard once every 6 months. (I think we may have been running around the battles of WWII with a scale, verifying Marine's weights.) I had surgery less than two months ago in which my abdomen was sliced open laparoscopically for a gynecological procedure.

I've been in the Corps for 13 years, enlisted and officer at 7 different ranks.

I've been running around in a sauna suit for a month. I haven't drank any alcohol/or anything with sugar in about three weeks, and also haven't had a carb since then either. 4 days ago I stopped eating solid foods completely. I took laxatives. Drank two bottles of magnesium citrate. I soaked in Epsom salts. I

foods completely. I took laxatives. Drank two bottles of magnesium citrate. I soaked in Epsom salts. I INJECTED Epsom salts. I spit in a bottle this morning, bringing me back to my high school wrestler days. I also made myself puke when I got to work just to ensure I was good to go for those last few ounces.

Many may and do say, "why don't you just tape?". The taping standards are from the 1980s and have proven to disproportionately discriminate against women and persons of color. (Look at the data, persons of color, especially African American women are forced out of the Corps at almost twice the rate of white males for weight issues). A recent NPS study showed that 70+ percent of women EVEN those WITHIN weight standards don't pass the female taping methods. This needs to be fixed, and it needs to be fixed now.

I taped myself for fun, the USMC way a few weeks ago. It showed I was damn near 40% body fat. We use a method that tapes the widest part of your hips, the narrowest part of your waist, then subtract the circumference of your neck. It is laughably inaccurate. My high speed scale tells me I am 26%, 2% lower than allowed for my age and gender.

Oh, and I made weight [redacted].

Special thanks to Coach [redacted] my teammates from high school. Wouldn't have been able to do it without the mental resiliency I learned as a [redacted].

(I do not advocate for these methods of weight loss, I speak up for those who can't or won't. These thoughts are my own and not those of the USMC)

Potential Impacts on Decisionmaking and Resilience

Beyond the impacts of disordered eating on individual marines' long-term mental and physical health, which may not fully materialize until a marine has left the service, there are potential performance impacts that may occur during service that need to be considered. Although research about these factors in the Marine Corps and the services is scarce, we can again look to the broader civilian population for discussion of what is known and where additional analysis is warranted. In this section, we discuss identified links

FIGURE 5.1—CONTINUED

Many of the responses to this post reflect agreement with the original poster's concerns about the challenges of meeting height and weight standards. Samples from these responses include the following:

- "I hated doing it trying to lose weight] to my body and it caused so much damage to my metabolism that it took 5 years to repair."
- "[T]his is one of the biggest reasons I'm getting out after this enlistment."
- "I do NOT miss having to dehydrate, starve, and damn near kill myself to make weight."
- "Every single weigh in that comes up I get anxious, afraid, and paranoid."
- "[I've] done every single one of those things you did numerous amounts of times."
- I'm literally forced to starve myself the week prior to weigh-ins and it's awful."

NOTE: The original post was made public in June 2021 by Capt Karen Holliday. Used with permission.

among nutrition, hydration, and high-level cognitive functioning, such as the kind required by stressful, high-pressure leadership decisionmaking.

It is important to understand that cognitive functioning, particularly at high levels, largely depends on internal physiological environments. The proper transmission of signals between brain neurons and the larger brain regions that govern complex mental and physical processes depend on adequate hydration and energy stores. Common behaviors employed by service members to conform with height and weight standards include fasting, dehydration, and similar calorie- and water-restricting means, which negatively influence cognitive functioning, making this a cause for concern.

The importance of proper hydration in cognitive functioning is often underemphasized. For example, short-term analyses found that healthy young adult men with low levels of hydration had slowed psychomotor-processing speed and poor attention and memory performance.[27] In long-term studies, dehydration was associated with an accelerated decline in well-being over time, along with trajectories of lower cognitive functioning and well-being. Although many long-term studies have been done in older adults, the mechanisms behind dehydration and cognitive decline suggest that dehydration may lead to the creation of defective proteins, which then may negatively affect cognitive functionality through impaired information processing. The continued dehydration and resulting production of these proteins may damage neurons and synaptic connections.[28]

Proper nutrition is also critical to cognitive functioning. Although the body can store energy sources in the form of glycogen in tissues and organs, the energy stores in the brain are small, especially considering the high level of glucose consumption and the consistent need for glucose to support functioning.[29] Low glucose levels can disrupt cognitive functioning, and supplying glucose through food or drink can improve memory for complex figures or attention-span motor functioning.[30]

Laboratory experiments have demonstrated that individuals who have eaten breakfast demonstrated better recall and verbal memory than those

[27] Rita Merhej, "Dehydration and Cognition: An Understated Relation," *International Journal of Health Governance*, Vol. 24, No. 1, 2019; and Julie A. Suhr, Jessica Hall, Stephen M. Patterson, and Rebecca Tong Niinistö, "The Relation of Hydration Status to Cognitive Performance in Healthy Older Adults," *International Journal of Psychophysiology*, Vol. 53, No. 2, July 2004.

[28] Konstantinos Mantantzis, Johanna Drewelies, Sandra Duezel, Elisabeth Steinhagen-Thiessen, Ilja Demuth, Gert G. Wagner, Ulman Lindenberger, and Denis Gerstorf, "Dehydration Predicts Longitudinal Decline in Cognitive Functioning and Well-Being Among Older Adults," *Psychology and Aging*, Vol. 35, No. 4, June 2020; and Adonis Sfera, Michael Cummings, and Carolina Osorio, "Dehydration and Cognition in Geriatrics: A Hydromolecular Hypothesis," *Frontiers in Molecular Biosciences*, Vol. 3, article 18, May 2016.

[29] David Benton, Pearl Y. Parker, and Rachael T. Donohoe, "The Supply of Glucose to the Brain and Cognitive Functioning," *Journal of Biosocial Science*, Vol. 28, No. 4, October 1996.

[30] David Benton and Pearl Y. Parker, "Breakfast, Blood Glucose, and Cognition," *American Journal of Clinical Nutrition*, Vol. 67, No. 4, April 1998; Carol A. Manning, J. L. Hall, Paul Ernest Gold, "Glucose Effects on Memory and Other Neuropsychological Tests in Elderly Humans," *Psychology and Science*, Vol. 1, No. 5, 1990.

who were fasting.[31] Such studies show that glucose fuels brain processing, especially when other factors, such as chronic fatigue, malnutrition, physical exertion, and the need to complete complex mental tasks, are in play. In one controlled experiment, 23 volunteers (young men and women with a mean age of 20 and 23, respectively, and all within normal weight ranges) were subjected to a restricted calorie condition, which was then compared with an ample caloric nutrition condition. The volunteers were then exposed to executive functioning tasks, such as rapidly switching attention from one task to another and making decisions, and given impulsivity, mood, and arousal tests following physical exertion. The intent was to understand how only two days of calorie deficits affect physical exertion and cognitive performance. Results revealed that, during exercise, calorie deprivation impaired performance on tasks of set-shifting and response inhibition but not risk-based decisionmaking. Calorie deprivation during exercise also impaired all aspects of mood assessed by the study—that is, it resulted in increased anger, lower vigor, greater fatigue, and increased confusion. Deprivation also led to increased tension and anxiety, depression and dejection, fatigue and inertia, confusion and bewilderment, increasing vigor and activity, and total mood disturbance. Additionally, levels of self-reported exertion increased during exercise. Most of the effects of calorie deprivation were observed on the second day, which was expected, because physiological and central nervous system effects of continuous calorie deprivation are additive over time.[32]

Past research has also focused on disordered eating behavior and long-term impacts on cognitive functioning. Studies examining effects of chronic caloric restriction using patients with long-term diagnosed disordered eating showed impairments in perceptual measures and nonverbal memory relative to healthy controls. This supports the idea that a cumulative effect of cognitive function is associated with disordered eating,

---

[31] Benton and Parker, 1998.

[32] Grace E. Giles, Caroline R. Mahoney, Christina Caruso, Asma S. Bukhari, Tracey J. Smith, Stefan M. Pasiakos, James P. McClung, and Harris R. Lieberman, "Two Days of Calorie Deprivation Impairs High Level Cognitive Processes, Mood, and Self-Reported Exertion During Aerobic Exercise: A Randomized Double-Blind, Placebo-Controlled Study," *Brain and Cognition*, Vol. 132, June 2019.

and that the number of years of experiencing caloric deficits is positively associated with impairments in cognition.[33]

Caloric deficits can also cause cognitive changes. Structural studies have shown that the duration of disordered eating was correlated with an individual's volume of gray matter, which holds neuronal cell bodies and governs muscle control and cognitive function. Compared with people with restored weights following disordered eating, brains scans showed a lower volume of gray matter at the low weight than at the restored weight. Importantly, the gray matter deficits improved with short-term weight restoration but did not fully recover.[34]

Looking specifically at AN, compared with control subjects, study participants with AN had enlarged ventricles, which suggests that gray matter decreases often follow neuronal death. AN participants performed more poorly than healthy control subjects across almost all the tested neuropsychological domains, such as those measuring verbal ability, cognitive efficiency, broad reading, broad math, and delayed verbal recall.[35] Recovered AN participants demonstrated no significant differences on these same domains and scores compared with healthy control participants. However, differences on all the above cognitive measures among AN participants, those in the healthy control group, and the weight-recovered group suggest that even six years after an initial diagnosis of AN, AN clinical participants still exhibited ventricular enlargements, commonly reported during the acute stages of the disorder.[36]

---

[33] Antoni Grau, Ernesto Magallón-Neri, Gustavo Faus, and Guillem Feixas, "Cognitive Impairment in Eating Disorder Patients of Short and Long-Term Duration: A Case-Control Study," *Neuropsychiatric Disease and Treatment*, Vol. 15, 2019.

[34] Christina A. Roberto, Laurel E. S. Mayer, Adam M. Brickman, Anna Barnes, Jordan Muraskin, Lok-Kin Yeung, Jason Steffener, Melissa Sy, Joy Hirsch, Yaakov Stern, and B. Timothy Walsh, "Brain Tissue Volume Changes Following Weight Gain in Adults with Anorexia Nervosa," *International Journal of Eating Disorders*, Vol. 44, No. 5, July 2011.

[35] Harold T. Chui, Bruce K. Christensen, Robert B. Zipursky, Blake A. Richards, M. Katherine Hanratty, Noor J. Kabani, David J. Mikulis, and Debra K. Katzman, "Cognitive Function and Brain Structure in Females with a History of Adolescent-Onset Anorexia Nervosa," *Pediatrics*, Vol. 122, No. 2, August 2008.

[36] Chui et al., 2008.

Given the cumulative effects of caloric deprivation on cognitive and physical performance we just outlined, the impacts of chronic deprivation on mental or physical performance of marines, particularly those in leadership positions and stressful situations, is cause for concern.[37]

Elite athletes are a parallel community that can provide some context. Although many laboratory studies have looked at clinical populations (e.g., those suffering from AN or BN), disordered eating remains very common in the athlete community. Up to 70 percent of elite athletes competing in weight class sports (male and female) are dieting and have some type of disordered eating pattern, with the goal of reducing weight before specific events or competitions.[38]

Female athletes often fall subject to the previously discussed female athlete triad. Many active women suffer from low bone density, chronic stress fractures, and menstrual irregularity, in particular amenorrhea, and all these factors increase this risk of injury. Moreover, these outcomes are highly connected to one another; past work has shown that amenorrheic athletes have two to four times greater risk of stress fractures than their eumenorrheic counterparts.[39] Although the effects may not be immediate after diagnosis of the triad, a decrease in peak skeletal bone-mineral density, along with skeletal demineralization occurring slowly over time, can lead to these conditions. Similarly, the resumption of menses does not resolve bone-mineral density issues immediately but starts the necessary rebuilding of bone to decrease the risk of future osteoporosis and fracture. Depending on the age of the patient, duration of the triad, and time to recovery, bone-mineral density may stabilize and even improve but not necessarily "catch up" to normal, age-appropriate bone-mineral density and could cause long-term risk to health and wellness of the individual and, in the context of the Marine Corps, the force.[40]

Female athletes suffering from the triad may not look like traditional patients with disordered eating. However, they often engage in a wide

[37] Giles et al., 2019.

[38] Nazem and Ackerman, 2012.

[39] Nazem and Ackerman, 2012.

[40] Nazem and Ackerman, 2012.

variety of harmful behaviors also exhibited in traditional patients, from food restriction to bingeing and purging or excessive exercise, to lose weight or maintain a thin physique. This may make the triad difficult to diagnose, because it does not meet the strict criteria for AN or BN that are listed in the DSM. Instead, disordered eating often manifests as part of the triad syndrome. Thus, changing traditional and truly antiquated standards of "physique" and wellness to recognize symptoms and allow for early diagnosis and treatment of problem conditions can help improve the health and wellness of female service members and the force as a whole.[41] Traditionally, athletes were screened for the triad by monitoring rates of fractures, weight change, eating behavior, amenorrhea, cardiac performance, and depression.[42] As health and wellness standards change for body composition, to be inclusive of more holistic measures of wellness and health, the ability to perform athletically and cognitively demanding tasks should be considered in both standard female military body composition and early screening and diagnosis of issues.

Disordered eating and body dysmorphia can be addressed through prevention. Superiors are often not cognizant or thoughtful about their impact on subordinates. One study showed that young female collegiate athletes who were told that they were overweight by coaches or other high-powered and respected individuals subsequently developed disordered eating behaviors, including daily implementation of self-induced vomiting, laxatives, diuretics, or diet pills, for at least a month to reduce or remain underweight. Thus, words and standards that female service members are repeatedly exposed to could have serious and potentially long-lasting side effects that are often not considered by authority figures who share and promote certain ideals.[43]

---

[41] Julie A. Hobart and Douglas R. Smucker, "The Female Athlete Triad," *American Family Physician*, Vol. 61, No. 11, June 2000.

[42] Hobart and Smucker, 2000.

[43] Ian M. Cockerill and Stephanie J. Quinton, "A Review of Pathogenic Weight-Control Behaviour Among Athletes: A Cause for Concern?" *Journal of the Institute of Health Education*, Vol. 33, No. 1, 1996; James C. Rosen, Nancy T. Silberg, and Janet Gross, "Eating Attitudes Test and Eating Disorders Inventory: Norms for Adolescent Girls and Boys," *Journal of Consulting and Clinical Psychology*, Vol. 56, No. 2, April 1988;

Additional Considerations

A closer examination of the policy and population of marines who exceed maximum height/weight and body-composition standards might find problematic behaviors within that group, because those marines in danger of failing to make weight attempt to lose weight or control weight in different ways. Additionally, those numbers alone—those who are controlling their weight or separated from the Corps for failing to comply with the policy—will provide information only about individuals who do not manage to make weight before being tested. (Because of the scope of this project, we were limited in our ability to collect such data, so we relied primarily on open-source material for these numbers. Data on marines separated for failing to meet height/weight standards are covered in the section on retention.) Potential effects of the policy may not be visible if the examination of impacts is limited to just those marines who exceed maximum standards. Marines who make weight—but by any means available—are also at risk of developing concerning behaviors, just as are those who fail to make weight. Marines who meet the height and weight standards are not subject to the greater scrutiny of their habits and behaviors as those who fall short are. In fact, given how the service prizes and praises peak physical fitness and appearance, marines who develop and maintain risky behaviors to conform to the policy and standards are not only hiding these behaviors and the potential impacts they bring, but they may be, concerningly, considered model marines.

Rather than examine only the characteristics and behaviors of marines on weight control or those separated from the service, it may be more appropriate to question whether marines who do meet height and weight standards suffer from problematic behaviors that underpin their apparent success. For example, what are marines who successfully conform to the published standards doing to make weight? Are there patterns to the behaviors that they adopt to make weight? What are the near- and long-term impacts of these behaviors? As existing research and recent commentary

---

and Lionel W. Rosen and David O. Hough, "Pathogenic Weight-Control Behaviors of Female College Gymnasts," *Physician and Sportsmedicine*, Vol. 16, No. 9, September 1988.

on this issue suggest, the BCMAP policy and its associated standards and career and cultural implications may shape individual marines' behavior in ways that can be detrimental to physical and mental health, both in the near and long term. These behaviors and their potential health impacts deserve deeper analysis. And, as we discuss in the next chapter, there also may be impacts on diversity, equity, and inclusion (DEI) and retention in the Marine Corps.

CHAPTER SIX

Impact of Body-Composition Standards on the Organization

In the previous chapter, we explored the impact of the BCMAP on individual behavior and health outcomes. But the impacts of BCMAP can be much broader, including at the organizational level. This chapter explores BCMAP's impacts on DEI and retention.

Diversity, Equity, and Inclusion

Research demonstrates that the development of BMI was centered on a White, European, male population.[1] Furthermore, the cut points associated with BMI tables used life insurance–policy standards created with data on mostly White policyholders. Despite these realities, the BMI standard and cut points are applied to more diverse populations. The World Health Organization has updated BMI cut points to accommodate people of Asian descent, but no similar adjustment in metrics have been made for Black and Latino populations.[2]

The circumference-based method of measurement can have implications for different demographic groups as well. Research has identified

---

[1] Stern, 2021.

[2] Rishi Caleyachetty, Thomas M. Barber, Nuredin Ibrahim Mohammed, Francesco P. Cappuccio, Rebecca Hardy, Rohini Mathur, Amitava Banerjee, and Paramijit Gill, "Ethnicity-Specific BMI Cutoffs for Obesity Based on Type 2 Diabetes Risk in England: A Population-Based Cohort Study," *The Lancet: Diabetes and Endocrinology*, Vol. 9, No. 7, May 11, 2021.

differences in fat distribution across different racial groups, ethnic groups, and genders, leading to inequitable outcomes across groups. For example, women tend to carry fat tissue in their hips, while men carry fat on their abdomen or trunk areas.[3] Additionally, Black women tend to carry fat tissue in their hips and upper thighs more than White women do.[4] For women, the tape test measures around the hip (greatest protrusion of the buttocks), which is where Black women generally have a substantially greater WHR than White counterparts.[5] Research that examined the body-composition measurements between Black people and White people in the general population concluded that there are differences in fat distribution between the two groups and that "because most equations that predict relative body fat were derived from predominantly White samples, biological variation between the races in these body-composition indexes has practical significance."[6] This difference in fat distribution among populations demonstrates that the circumference-based method of measurement is not optimized to account for body makeup of diverse racial and ethnic groups.

The use of these standards and measurements can negatively affect people of color in the Marine Corps. According to a recent analysis by the

---

[3] Terry T. K. Huang, Maria S. Johnson, Reinaldo Figueroa-Colon, James H. Dwyer, and Michael I. Goran, "Growth of Visceral Fat, Subcutaneous Abdominal Fat, and Total Body Fat in Children," *Obesity Research*, Vol. 9, No. 5, May 2001; and Peter T. Katzmarzyk, George A. Bray, Frank L. Greenway, William D. Johnson, Robert L. Newton, Jr., Eric Ravussin, Donna H. Ryan, Steven R. Smith, and Claude Bouchard, "Racial Differences in Abdominal Depot-Specific Adiposity in White and African American Adults," *American Journal of Clinical Nutrition*, Vol. 91, No. 1, January 2010.

[4] Juhua Luo, Michael Hendryx, Deepika Laddu, Lawrence S. Phillips, Rowan Chlebowski, Erin S. LeBlanc, David B. Allison, Dorothy A. Nelson, Yueyao Li, Milagros C. Rosal, Marcia L. Stefanik, and JoAnn E. Manson, "Racial and Ethnic Differences in Anthropometric Measures as Risk Factors for Diabetes," *Diabetes Care*, Vol. 42, No. 1, January 2019.

[5] Valonne Ehrhardt, "Assessing Physical and Combat Readiness: Abandon the Marine Corps Body Composition Program," thesis, Quantico, Va.: Naval Postgraduate School, 2021.

[6] Dale R. Wagner and Vivian H. Heyward, "Measures of Body Composition in Blacks and Whites: A Comparative Review," *American Journal of Clinical Nutrition*, Vol. 71, No. 6, June 2000.

Marine Corps Human Performance Branch, women who are Black or of Hawaiian/Pacific Islander descent have the highest rates of being overweight (8.3 percent and 7.2 percent, respectively).[7] Black and Hispanic women also have the highest rate of being overfat—at 2.7 percent and 2.5 percent, respectively, compared with 2.2 percent for all female marines.[8] These Marine Corps Human Performance Branch statistics come from a Naval Postgraduate School thesis published earlier this year, and we were unable to independently verify the statistics for this project because of the limited scope. Additionally, administrative discharges related to body composition for these groups are higher. In 2014, 9 percent of female marine discharges were for body fat–testing failures, compared with 7 percent for male marines.[9] Women already are already a minority within the force (8 percent of officers, 9 percent of enlisted as of 2020), so the higher rate of discharges may negatively affect minority retention and promotion.[10] Because the Marine Corps places heavy emphasis on appearance, the perception that certain minority groups fail to meet BCMAP standards may contribute to perpetuating gender and racial biases in the service.

Retention

Our analysis of the literature found that there is a significant gap in research about the impacts of the BCP on retention. Data collection related to body composition and attrition varies by service and is not always accurate. Tracking data related to physical fitness, weight for height, and body fat percentage is done at the service level and is not consistent across DoD.[11] Studies that focus on issues related to body composition among the force often use survey data that rely heavily on self-reported responses, which may not

---

[7] Ehrhardt, 2021.

[8] Ehrhardt, 2021. *Overweight* refers to service members exceeding the service's height and weight standard, and *overfat* refers to exceeding the service's body standard as measured by circumference-based method (DoDI 1308.3).

[9] Ehrhardt, 2021.

[10] Council on Foreign Relations, "Demographics of the U.S. Military," webpage, July 13, 2020.

[11] Defense Health Board, 2013.

correspond with measured data. Other studies use medical administrative data, where medical codes related to obesity may be applied incorrectly, if at all. Therefore, the precise number of affected individuals may not be reflected in the data. This lack of uniform data collection on force fitness leads to gaps in understanding the breadth of issues the force faces.

Primarily, research about the relationship between body composition and retention has focused on accession and first-term enlistments to determine if obesity and/or overweightness is a predictor of attrition. Studies demonstrate that, for recruits who exceed height/weight standards prior to joining the military and either receive a waiver or meet standards later, "80% left the military before completing their first term of enlistment but after the expenditure of training costs."[12] Most of the research is framed from a cost perspective, indicating that the service is concerned about sinking costs into training without a return on investment.

Although the research focuses on retaining service members at the beginning of their career, to ensure return on expended costs, there has been limited research about the impact of overweight medical diagnoses on remaining time in service past the initial training period. Research demonstrates that military members diagnosed as obese or overweight have shorter service time in the near term compared with populations who do not receive a diagnosis. One study reviewed data from the Armed Forces Health Surveillance Center, which tracks population-based data on attrition accounting for health and weight factors. Using time in service following failure to meet body-composition standards as a proxy for time of discharge, the center was able to estimate impacts on retention. The center found that, for a four-year period from 2006 to 2010, "the durations of service for those with an overweight-related diagnosis were 18 months shorter for obese individuals and 9 months shorter for overweight individuals than for those not receiving such diagnoses."[13] Data from the same study showed that, after three years, there was no impact on retention, because those who were diagnosed as overweight remained just as likely to be retained by the service as those who were not diagnosed

[12] Erin Tompkins, *Obesity in the United States and Effects on Military Recruiting*, Washington, D.C.: Congressional Research Service, December 22, 2020.

[13] Defense Health Board, 2013.

as overweight. Of the populations included in the study, Hispanic and Black non-Hispanic personnel had the shortest durations of service following a diagnosis of overweight and, of the services, the Marine Corps had the shortest duration of service following a diagnosis.[14] The report covers those individuals in the active and reserve forces who received diagnoses during the period of review, and the author estimates that the number of individuals affected is underrepresented.

Because of the scope of this project, we were unable to independently access data related to service members and body-composition statistics. Therefore, we relied on open-source data to understand the totality of the problem. Annual data about number of service members who separate from the service because of body-composition failures are sporadic and spotty. Other research has raised concerns about the accuracy of the data resulting from inconsistent data-collection and reporting requirements by service.[15] That being said, there has been recent media coverage of the number of service members who are forced out because of not making height and weight requirements. For the Marine Corps, discharges related to BCP and/or the PFA numbered 92 in 2010, 186 in 2011, and 132 in 2012.[16] More recent numbers are not available.

Although the number of separations resulting from height-and-weight-requirement failures is numerically small, there is potentially a larger portion of the service that self-selects out to prevent failing and/or engages in unhealthy behaviors to maintain standards. Anecdotally, the Army has stated that "typically, subject officers will resign prior to forced separation."[17] Similarly, research has found that, in the Army and Marine Corps, women report negative career paths when they fail a height-weight measurements, even if their body fat is within

---

[14] Armed Forces Health Surveillance Center, 2008.

[15] U.S. General Accounting Office, *Military Attrition: Better Data, Coupled with Policy Changes, Could Help the Services Reduce Early Separations*, report to the chairman and the ranking minority member, Subcommittee on Personnel, Committee on Armed Services, U.S. Senate, Washington, D.C., GAO/NSIAD-98-213, September 1998.

[16] "Experts: Tape Test Has Huge Margin of Error," *Military Times*, May 21, 2013; and Defense Health Board, 2013.

[17] Defense Health Board, 2013.

body-composition standards.[18] Therefore, although failure to make standards may not be the reason for separation, BCP may be a contributing factor.

Post-service impacts are another area for research. Studies have shown that military members increase weight gain around the time discharge.[19] For the period between discharge to three years post-discharge, military veterans show significant weight gain. Hypotheses for this weight gain are increased food consumption with an associated decrease in activity, inability to break eating patterns learned in the service, food insecurity, and eating to compensate for stress related to military experiences.[20] These findings indicate that service members are at risk for unhealthy eating-related behaviors during the time of separation and immediately following, and they echo the increased risks of other health consequences that military members are already subject to because of the nature of military life.

To understand the totality of the issue, further research should include examining reasons that service members leave the force and whether their decisions are influenced by the BCP. Critically, this research should include an assessment of why members of diverse demographic groups, particularly women of color, leave the force. This question could be tracked through exit interviews or annual health screens to ensure widest reach. We also recommend a quantitative analysis of the force to explore what parts of the military population are within 1–2 percent of the height and weight standards and how that population breaks down across demographic groups. This would help decisionmakers understand the needs and composition of the community "on the bubble" and can help leaders understand any inequitable impacts of the BCMAP. Conducting focus groups with service members to ask them how BCP influences their decision to remain in the force could also be beneficial, particularly if diverse representation is purposely sought for focus groups. There is an opportunity to reframe the narrative from one

---

[18] McNulty, 2001.

[19] Alyson J. Littman, Isabel G. Jacobson, Edward J. Boyko, Teresa Powell, and Tyler C. Smith, for the Millennium Cohort Study Team, "Weight Change Follow U.S. Military Service," *International Journal of Obesity*, Vol. 37, No. 2, February 2013.

[20] Defense Health Board, 2013.

focused on obesity and its cost to one that places overall health and wellness at the center.

Summary

The current manifestation and implementation of the BCMAP may be inequitable across different demographic groups of marines and may have impacts on retention, particularly retention within different groups. As of this writing, however, research about potential impacts of the policy on DEI in the force and associated behaviors is virtually nonexistent, and awareness of how the BCMAP affects retention is restricted to the publication of discharge numbers related to the policy, which can be one-dimensional. Additional research is needed to understand the elevated risks marines face, particularly female marines and marines of color, and the potential impacts of those behaviors on the health of marines and the force as a whole.

CHAPTER SEVEN

Findings and Recommendations

Our research aimed to build understanding of the BCMAP and its impacts along four key research subject areas: (1) the existing policy and its scientific foundations, (2) the impacts of body-composition standards on individual health choices, (3) the impacts of these health choices on the short- and long-term mental and physical health of personnel, and (4) the impacts on the institution. The research was also designed to provide recommendations for policy change and future research to be considered. In this chapter, we provide our findings, recommendations for potential policy change, and recommendations for future research and exploration.

Findings

The BCMAP and associated standards exist, per the policy, to ensure that marines are both fit and healthy. Both aspects are integral parts of the BCP. However, our research findings present a conflict between these reasons. We found that the implementation of the policy, specifically through the standards it codifies, places it at odds with the intent to ensure that marines are both fit and healthy.

Specifically, we found that the BCMAP and its implementation may be inequitable across demographic groups, may be unnecessarily risking the health of individual marines and the force as a whole, and may also be negatively affecting retention, particularly across all demographic groups. By directly linking a failure to maintain strict height and weight standards—specifically standards developed using an unrepresentative group of people on top of the addition of increased requirements for the development of muscle mass—to an individual's leadership qualities and career prospects, the BCMAP may make marines more likely to adopt unhealthy behaviors to conform to standards.

These behaviors are associated with eating disorders, including self-induced vomiting, laxative and diet pill use, sauna and diuretic use, excessive exercise, and fasting. Existing research documents significantly elevated rates of these behaviors among marines, along with associated short- and long-term mental and physical health impacts, including cognitive functioning impairment, reproductive and skeletal problems, depression, and suicide risk. These behaviors can affect the health of the force and retention. As noted earlier, it is not enough to look only at eating disorder diagnosis rates, which already place marines at an elevated risk. Because of the stigma associated with disordered eating and the fitness-embracing culture of the Marine Corps, disordered eating behaviors may be more prevalent than diagnosis rates suggest.

Furthermore, as just explained, marines, like all service members, are at elevated risk for different kinds of trauma. Trauma places individuals at greater risk of disordered eating behaviors and the breadth of mental and physical comorbidities associated with those behaviors. Because women are already at increased risk of disordered eating because of MST, potential impacts of the BCMAP may be piling on even greater risk for women.

Research Recommendations

Given these findings, we recommend that the Marine Corps pursue an overall systems approach to fully understand and address the deficiencies in the BCMAP, develop a more health-focused policy, and mitigate any negative impacts from the existing BCMAP. This approach should encompass the following:[1]

1. Clearly define the objective of the policy (independent of what the original objective may have been).

[1] E. S. Quade, *The Systems Approach and Public Policy*, Santa Monica, Calif.: RAND Corporation, P-4053, 1969.

2. Thoroughly investigate possible alternatives for feasibility, risk, and cost.
3. Compare alternatives in terms of outcomes.
4. Assess and mitigate any potential negative impacts of the existing BCMAP.

As part of this process, we recommend that Marine Corps leaders consider the steps we outline in the next section, which are both actionable and informative, as they help the institution identify a more appropriate policy that balances body-composition requirements for health and performance equitably for *all* marines of every demographic group.

Policy Recommendations

We recommend the following actions that the Marine Corps can take in the short term:

1. Consider pausing all height and weight and body-composition measurements while the Corps considers the following steps and assesses impacts. This includes pausing the recording of height and weight and body-composition measurements on relevant reports and the pursuit of career-affecting steps for those who exceed maximum height and weight and tape measurements. Our research demonstrates that marines are at higher risk of developing disordered eating behaviors than their civilian counterparts, and that risk is driven in part by the substance and implementation of the BCMAP. We believe that the safety of marines calls for a pause as other measurement standards and methods are explored. This pause can remove the risk to marines caused by the policy.
2. The Marine Corps should comprehensively and systematically reevaluate whether height and weight are still necessary requirements for marines—and if they are as representative of overall fitness and health as they are considered to be per the BCMAP.
   a. This determination should include considering whether removing height and weight and body-composition measurements from health and fitness assessments would

affect individuals and/or the institution and, if so, how. Specifically, this evaluation should include a consideration of potential inequitable impacts of existing height and weight and body-composition measurements to ensure that policy equity is a cornerstone.

b. If it is determined that height and weight and body composition should remain a requirement, even if only in specific MOSs, the Corps should undertake a comprehensive analysis to determine the following:
   i. Are the standards appropriate, given the increased requirements to build muscle mass and associated strength? This analysis should include consideration of what the appropriate standards should be across all demographic groups, along with consideration of how individuals across demographic groups build muscle and strength.
   ii. Are the measurement methods appropriate? Although no method appears to be both practical for field use and free of error, we recommend that the Marine Corps explore ways to decrease errors introduced by simpler methods or acquire the means to more accurately measure body composition in marines. This analysis should include consideration of the variation in accuracy of body-composition measurement methods across race, gender, and ethnic lines.

3. Reassess the need to include verbiage in the BCMAP that directly links weight and appearance to the leadership, discipline, and character of marines. Although appearance is an important functional part of Marine Corps culture, the emphasis to "make weight" can result in unhealthy behaviors and lead to shame. As discussed throughout this report, cultures that emphasize appearance and weight place members at higher risk of developing disordered eating behavior. Understanding how this cultural norm evolved in the Marine Corps and coalesced is important to determine if the norm remains a foundational value. We recommend that the Marine Corps clarify and balance the tension between

acknowledging cultural norms and ensuring the health and well-being of the force.

4. Develop and implement a BCP that directly grapples with the contradictory nature of the existing program—the trade-offs between thinness and performance that marines often struggle with. A new program should delineate requirements for both health and performance, and the program should be further assessed to ensure that it is equitably applied to marines across demographic groups. This assessment should also consider how the health and fitness of pregnant and postpartum women should be considered within this paradigm. We recommend that the Marine Corps conduct a study to identify marines who are making weight and whose behaviors blend in, along with those who exceed the standards.
5. Beyond the revision and adjustment of the policy itself, we recommend that the Marine Corps explore the risk of disordered eating behavior and the long-term physical and mental health impacts on marines. We suggest a three-pronged exploration:
    a. Destigmatize eating disorders and build awareness of the prevalence of disordered eating behavior, particularly near weigh-in periods. Training on disordered eating, risks, symptoms, and impacts for leaders and health care providers is a start. This can also include ensuring that marines are aware of unhealthy, risky behaviors; how they manifest; and their long-term impacts. Training should also include broader dissemination of information about how marines can get help for individuals showing signs of risky or unhealthy behaviors.
    b. Relatedly, develop a purposeful education and communication strategy to accompany any policy changes. An education and communication strategy that emphasizes health and performance can target culture and help mitigate lasting effects of the existing policy. Because, as just noted, cultures that emphasize appearance and weight can place members at higher risk of developing unhealthy behaviors, simply changing the policy alone may not be enough to lower the risk to marines.

c. Increase and regularly screen for and prevent disordered eating symptoms. This can potentially be done as part of annual physicals, preventative health assessments, and other regular health care touchpoints. This screening can help leaders and providers catch risky behavior earlier and enable intervention. Additionally, this can help the Corps collect and analyze data to better understand the scope and scale of the problem.

Recommendations for Additional Research

Finally, we found the absence of substantive research about how diverse groups are potentially affected by the BCMAP, existing standards and measurement methods, and disordered eating behavior to be problematic. The policy affects marines in ways that can follow them for years, so understanding how diverse demographic groups are affected is critical to building awareness and understanding of what those impacts are. The recommendations that we proposed are first steps, but we recommend additional research about how service members across DoD are affected by DoD and service policies, how veterans are affected by longer-term disordered eating behaviors and associated mental and physical health comorbidities, and how these two factors may affect retention and readiness as a whole across DoD.

We recommended additional research in these areas:

- Understand who may be on the cusp of failing standards and therefore may be more at risk for harmful behaviors. As mentioned earlier, the marines who fail to make standards are at risk of harmful behaviors. However, those who meet the standard are at risk as well, except they avoid scrutiny. The analysis should also include a broader survey or analysis of as large a population of marines, particularly marines of different demographic groups, as possible.
- Broadly collect and continue to analyze data. From the screening and analysis listed earlier in this chapter to outreach to the Marine Corps veteran community, a broader analysis of those potentially affected by the BCMAP and how those impacts manifest can identify

individuals who are still at risk of harm today. This data collection and analysis should also include transgender marines to identify how binary gender standards may affect them and what healthy standards could be. We recommend including the VA in this outreach and analysis to ensure that subjects receive appropriate care moving forward.

- Assess whether and how Marine Corps culture may have coalesced around the existing BCMAP. As noted earlier in this chapter, the verbiage in the existing BCMAP directly links weight and appearance to leadership, discipline, and character, and cultures that emphasize appearance and weight place members at higher risk of developing unhealthy behaviors. If the culture of the Marine Corps falls into this category, policy changes will need to be accompanied by a purposeful education and communication strategy to ensure that culture changes accompany policy shifts.
- Understand the totality of the issue by including more research about reasons service members leave the force and whether their decisions are influenced by the BCP. Critically, this research should include assessments of why members of diverse demographic groups, particularly women of color, leave the force.
- Conduct more research that explores the impact of the body-composition policy on military readiness and the lethality of the force. Beyond what has been outlined here, it is possible that this policy has lasting impacts on force readiness. We found this to be an area that has not been fully explored.

Abbreviations

ACFT	Army Combat Fitness Test
ADP	air displacement plethysmography
AN	anorexia nervosa
BCA	body-composition assessment
BCMAP	Body Composition Military Appearance Program
BCP	body-composition program
BED	binge-eating disorder
BIA	bioelectric impedance analysis
BMI	body mass index
BN	bulimia nervosa
CDC	Centers for Disease Control and Prevention
CFT	Combat Fitness Test
DEI	diversity, equity, and inclusion
DEXA	dual energy X-ray absorptiometry
DoD	U.S. Department of Defense
DoDI	Department of Defense Instruction
DSM	Diagnostic and Statistical Manual of Mental Disorders
EDNOS	eating disorder not otherwise specified
MCO	Marine Corps Order
MOS	military occupational specialty
MST	military sexual trauma
PFA	physical fitness assessment
PFT	physical fitness test
PTSD	posttraumatic stress disorder
VA	U.S. Department of Veterans Affairs
WC	waist circumference
WHR	waist-to-hip ratio

References

Air Force Manual 36-2905, *Air Force Physical Fitness Program*, Washington, D.C.: Secretary of the Air Force, December 11, 2020. As of September 29, 2021: https://www.afpc.af.mil/Portals/70/documents/FITNESS/afman36-2905.pdf?ver=e2q87ionZmRdxK0rm1SWEQ%3D%3D

American Psychiatric Association, "What Are Eating Disorders?" webpage, March 2021. As of May 21, 2021: https://www.psychiatry.org/patients-families/eating-disorders/what-are-eating-disorders

Archer, Emerald M., "The Power of Gendered Stereotypes in the U.S. Marine Corps," *Armed Forces and Society*, Vol. 39, No. 2, 2013, pp. 359–391.

Armed Forces Health Surveillance Center, "Diagnoses of Overweight/Obesity, Active Component, U.S. Armed Forces, 1998–2010," *Medical Surveillance Monthly Report*, Vol. 18, No. 1, January 2008, pp. 7–11. As of October 11, 2021: https://health.mil/Reference-Center/Reports/2011/01/01/Medical-Surveillance-Monthly-Report-Volume-18-Number-1

Army Regulation 600-9, *The Army Weight Control Program*, Washington, D.C.: Headquarters, Department of the Army, November 27, 2006. As of September 24, 2021: https://dmna.ny.gov/forms/ar600-9.pdf

Army Regulation 600–9, *The Army Body Composition Program*, Washington, D.C.: Headquarters, Department of the Army, July 16, 2019. As of September 29, 2021: https://armypubs.army.mil/epubs/DR_pubs/DR_a/pdf/web/ARN7779_AR600-9_FINAL.pdf

Bakalar, Jennifer L., Marissa Barmine, Lindsay Druskin, Cara H. Olsen, Jeffrey Quinlan, Tracy Sbrocco, and Marian Tanofsky-Kraff, "Childhood Adverse Life Events, Disordered Eating, and Body Mass Index in U.S. Military Service Members," *International Journal of Eating Disorders*, Vol. 51, No. 5, May 2018, pp. 465–469.

Bartlett, Brooke A., and Karen S. Mitchell, "Eating Disorders in Military and Veteran Men and Women: A Systematic Review," *International Journal of Eating Disorders*, Vol. 48, No. 8, December 2015, pp. 1057–1069.

Benton, David, and Pearl Y. Parker, "Breakfast, Blood Glucose, and Cognition," *American Journal of Clinical Nutrition*, Vol. 67, No. 4, April 1998, pp. 772S–778S.

Benton, David, Pearl Y. Parker, and Rachael T. Donohoe. "The Supply of Glucose to the Brain and Cognitive Functioning," *Journal of Biosocial Science*, Vol. 28, No. 4, October 1996, pp. 463–479.

Berkman, Nancy D., Kathleen N. Lohr, and Cynthia M. Bulik, "Outcomes of Eating Disorders: A Systematic Review of the Literature," *International Journal of Eating Disorders*, Vol. 40, No. 4, May 2007, pp. 293–309.

Bodell, Lindsay, Katherine Jean Forney, Pamela Keel, Peter Gutierrez, and Thomas E. Joiner, "Consequences of Making Weight: A Review of Eating Disorder Symptoms and Diagnoses in the United States Military," *Clinical Psychology*, Vol. 21, No. 4, 2014, pp. 398–409.

Borga, Magnus, Janne West, Jimmy D. Bell, Nicholas C. Harvey, Thobias Romu, Steven B. Heymsfield, and Olof Dahlqvist Leinhard, "Advanced Body Composition Assessment: From Body Mass Index to Body Composition Profiling," *Journal of Investigative Medicine*, Vol. 66, No. 5, June 2018, pp. 1–9.

Britzky, Haley, "How the Army Combat Fitness Test Exposes the Military's Unhealthy Focus on 'Making Weight,'" *Task and Purpose*, March 9, 2011. As of June 3, 2021:
https://taskandpurpose.com/news/acft-army-height-weight-standards/

Britzky, Haley, "'We Are All Suffering in Silence'—Inside the US Military's Pervasive Culture of Eating Disorders," *Task and Purpose*, August 2, 2021. As of December 20, 2021:
https://taskandpurpose.com/news/military-eating-disorders/

Brown, Elise C., Tamara Hew-Butler, Charles R. C. Marks, Scotty J. Butcher, and Myung D. Choi, "The Impact of Different High-Intensity Interval Training Protocols on Body Composition and Physical Fitness in Healthy Young Adult Females," *BioResearch Open Access*, Vol. 7.1, 2018. As of March 15, 2021:
https://www.liebertpub.com/doi/pdf/10.1089/biores.2018.0032

Caleyachetty, Rishi, Thomas M. Barber, Nuredin Ibrahim Mohammed, Francesco P. Cappuccio, Rebecca Hardy, Rohini Mathur, Amitava Banerjee, and Paramjit Gill, "Ethnicity-Specific BMI Cutoffs for Obesity Based on Type 2 Diabetes Risk in England: A Population-Based Cohort Study," *The Lancet: Diabetes and Endocrinology*, Vol. 9, No. 7, May 11, 2021, pp. 419–426.

Centers for Disease Control and Prevention, "About Adult BMI," webpage, August 27, 2021. As of June 3, 2021:
https://www.cdc.gov/healthyweight/assessing/bmi/adult_bmi/index.html

Chui, Harold T., Bruce K. Christensen, Robert B. Zipursky, Blake A. Richards, M. Katherine Hanratty, Noor J. Kabani, David J. Mikulis, and Debra K. Katzman, "Cognitive Function and Brain Structure in Females with a History of Adolescent-Onset Anorexia Nervosa," *Pediatrics*, Vol. 122, No. 2, August 2008, pp. e426–e437.

Cobb, Erin L., Angela L. Lamson, Coral Steffey, Alexander M. Schoemann, and Katharine W. Didericksen, "Disordered Eating and Military Populations: Understanding the Role of Adverse Childhood Experiences," *Journal of Military, Veteran and Family Health*, Vol. 6, No. 1, May 2020, pp. 70–82.

Cockerill, Ian M., and Stephanie J. Quinton, "A Review of Pathogenic Weight-Control Behaviour Among Athletes: A Cause for Concern?" *Journal of the Institute of Health Education*, Vol. 33, No. 1, 1996, pp. 13–15.

Council on Foreign Relations editors, "Demographics of the U.S. Military," webpage, July 13, 2020. As of June 20, 2021:
https://www.cfr.org/backgrounder/demographics-us-military

Defense Advisory Committee on Women in the Services, *2019 Annual Report*, November 13, 2019. As of July 29, 2021:
https://dacowits.defense.gov/Portals/48/Documents/Reports/2019/Annual%20Report/DACOWITS%202019.pdf?ver=2020-03-27-095608-557

Defense Health Board, *Implications of Trends in Obesity and Overweight for the Department of Defense*, Falls Church, Va., November 22, 2013. As of June 22, 2021:
https://health.mil/Reference-Center/Reports/2013/11/22/DHB-Implications-of-Trends-in-Obesity-and-Overweight-for-the-DoD-Fit-to-fight-fit-for-life

Department of Defense Directive 1308.1, *DoD Physical Fitness and Body Fat Program*, Washington, D.C.: U.S. Department of Defense, June 30, 2004. As of October 19, 2021:
https://www.esd.whs.mil/Portals/54/Documents/DD/issuances/dodd/130801p.pdf

Department of Defense Instruction 1308.3, *DoD Physical Fitness and Body Fat Programs Procedures*, Washington, D.C.: U.S. Department of Defense, November 5, 2002. As of September 29, 2021:
https://www.esd.whs.mil/Portals/54/Documents/DD/issuances/dodi/130803p.pdf

DoDI—*See* Department of Defense Instruction.

Donalson, Rosemary, *Disordered Eating in Female Veterans with Military Trauma*, dissertation, San Francisco, Calif.: California Institute of Integral Studies, 2016. As of September 24, 2021:
https://www.proquest.com/dissertations-theses/disordered-eating-female-veterans-with-military/docview/1868839424/se-2?accountid=25333

Duren, Dana L., Richard J. Sherwood, Stefan A. Czerwinski, Miryoung Lee, Audrey C. Choh, Roger M. Siervogel, and Wm. Camera Chumlea, "Body Composition Methods: Comparison and Interpretation," *Journal of Diabetes Science and Technology*, Vol. 2, No. 6, 2008, pp. 1139–1146.

Ehrhardt, Valonne, "Assessing Physical and Combat Readiness: Abandon the Marine Corps Body Composition Program," thesis, Quantico, Va.: Naval Postgraduate School, January 2021.

"Experts: Tape Test Has Huge Margin of Error," *Military Times*, May 21, 2013. As of June 3, 2021:
https://www.militarytimes.com/off-duty/military-fitness/2013/05/21/experts-tape-test-has-huge-margin-of-error/

Fairweather-Schmidt, A. Kate, Christina Lee, and Tracey D. Wade, "A Longitudinal Study of Midage Women with Indicators of Disordered Eating," *Developmental Psychology*, Vol. 51, No. 5, 2015, pp. 722–729.

"Feeding and Eating Disorders," American Psychiatric Association, 2013. As of June 3, 2021:
https://www.psychiatry.org/File%20Library/Psychiatrists/Practice/DSM/APA_DSM-5-Eating-Disorders.pdf

Forman-Hoffman, Valerie L., Michelle Mengeling, Brenda M. Booth, James Torner, and Anne G. Sadler, "Eating Disorders, Post-Traumatic Stress, and Sexual Trauma in Women Veterans," *Military Medicine*, Vol. 177, No. 10, October 2012, pp. 1161–1168.

Giles, Grace E., Caroline R. Mahoney, Christina Caruso, Asma S. Bukhari, Tracey J. Smith, Stefan M. Pasiakos, James P. McClung, and Harris R. Lieberman, "Two Days of Calorie Deprivation Impairs High Level Cognitive Processes, Mood, and Self-Reported Exertion During Aerobic Exercise: A Randomized Double-Blind, Placebo-Controlled Study," *Brain and Cognition*, Vol. 132, June 2019, pp. 33–40.

Grau, Antoni, Ernesto Magallón-Neri, Gustavo Faus, and Guillem Feixas, "Cognitive Impairment in Eating Disorder Patients of Short and Long-Term Duration: A Case-Control Study," *Neuropsychiatric Disease and Treatment*, Vol. 15, 2019, p. 1329–1341.

Harkins, Gina, "Female Marines Who Called Out the Corps Commend New Postpartum Policy," *Military.com*, February 11, 2021. As of December 22, 2021:
https://www.military.com/daily-news/2021/02/11/female-marines-who-called-out-corps-commend-new-postpartum-policy.html

Himmerich, Hubertus, Carol Kan, Katie Au, and Janet Treasure, "Pharmacological Treatment of Eating Disorders, Comorbid Mental Health Problems, Malnutrition, and Physical Health Consequences," *Pharmacology and Therapeutics*, Vol. 217, January 2021, p. 107667.

Hobart, Julie A., and Douglas R. Smucker, "The Female Athlete Triad," *American Family Physician*, Vol. 61, No. 11, June 2000, pp. 3357–3364.

Hogan, Kerry, *Review of the Current Body Fat Taping Method and Its Importance in Ascertaining Fitness Levels in the United States Marine Corps*, dissertation, Monterey, Calif.: Naval Postgraduate School, 2015. As of September 24, 2021:
http://hdl.handle.net/10945/45876

Huang, Terry T.-K., Maria S. Johnson, Reinaldo Figueroa-Colon, James H. Dwyer, and Michael I. Goran, "Growth of Visceral Fat, Subcutaneous Abdominal Fat, and Total Body Fat in Children," *Obesity Research*, Vol. 9, No. 5, May 2001, pp. 283–289.

Huston, J. C., A. R. Grillo, K. M. Iverson, K. S. Mitchell, and VA Boston Healthcare System, "Associations Between Disordered Eating and Intimate Partner Violence Mediated by Depression and Posttraumatic Stress Disorder Symptoms in a Female Veteran Sample," *General Hospital Psychiatry*, Vol. 58, May–June 2019, pp. 77–82.

Institute of Medicine, *Assessing Readiness in Military Women: The Relationship of Body, Composition, Nutrition, and Health*, Washington, D.C.: National Academies Press, 1998. As of September 24, 2021:
https://www.nap.edu/catalog/6104
/assessing-readiness-in-military-women-the-relationship-of-body-composition

Kärkkäinen, Ulla, Linda Mustelin, Anu Raevuori, Jaakko Kaprio, and Anna Keski-Rahkonen, "Do Disordered Eating Behaviours Have Long-Term Health-Related Consequences?" *European Eating Disorders Review*, Vol. 26, No. 1, January 2018, pp. 22–28.

Katzmarzyk, Peter T., George A. Bray, Frank L. Greenway, William D. Johnson, Robert L. Newton, Jr., Eric Ravussin, Donna H. Ryan, Steven R. Smith, and Claude Bouchard, "Racial Differences in Abdominal Depot-Specific Adiposity in White and African American Adults," *American Journal of Clinical Nutrition*, Vol. 91, No. 1, January 2010, pp. 7–15.

Kime, Patricia, "Congress Wants the Pentagon to Expand Coverage for Troops' Eating Disorder Treatments," *Military.com*, August 12, 2020. As of June 3, 2021:
https://www.military.com/daily-news/2020/08/12/congress-wants-pentagon
-expand-coverage-troops-eating-disorder-treatments.html

Kitzinger, H. B., and B. Karle, *The Epidemiology of Obesity*, Vol. 45, Vienna, Austria: Springer Vienna, 2013.

Kuriyan, Rebecca, "Body Composition Techniques," *Indian Journal of Medical Research*, Vol. 148, No. 5, 2018, pp. 648–658.

Lauder, Tamara D., Marc V. Williams, Carol S. Campbell, Gary Davis, Richard Sherman, and Elizabeth Pulos, "The Female Athlete Triad: Prevalence in Military Women," *Military Medicine*, Vol. 164, No. 9, September 1999, pp. 630–635.

Littman, Alyson J., Isabel G. Jacobson, Edward J. Boyko, Teresa Powell, and Tyler C. Smith, for the Millennium Cohort Study Team, "Weight Change Follow U.S. Military Service," *International Journal of Obesity*, Vol. 37, No. 2, February 2013, pp. 244–253.

Luo, Juhua, Michael Hendryx, Deepika Laddu, Lawrence S. Phillips, Rowan Chlebowski, Erin S. LeBlanc, David B. Allison, Dorothy A. Nelson, Yueyao Li, Milagros C. Rosal, Marcia L. Stefanik, and JoAnn E. Manson, "Racial and Ethnic Differences in Anthropometric Measures as Risk Factors for Diabetes," *Diabetes Care*, Vol. 42, No. 1, January 2019, pp. 126–133.

Manning, Carol A., J. L. Hall, and Paul Ernest Gold, "Glucose Effects on Memory and Other Neuropsychological Tests in Elderly Humans," *Psychological Science*, Vol. 1, No. 5, 1990, pp. 307–311.

Mantantzis, Konstantinos, Johanna Drewelies, Sandra Duezel, Elisabeth Steinhagen-Thiessen, Ilja Demuth, Gert G. Wagner, Ulman Lindenberger, and Denis Gerstorf, "Dehydration Predicts Longitudinal Decline in Cognitive Functioning and Well-Being Among Older Adults," *Psychology and Aging*, Vol. 35, No. 4, June 2020, pp. 517–528.

Marine Corps Order 6100.3C, *Physical Fitness,* Washington, D.C.: Commandant of the Marine Corps, 1956.

Marine Corps Order 6100.3G, *Physical Fitness, Weight Control and Military Appearance,* Washington, D.C.: Commandant of the Marine Corps, September 23, 1975.

Marine Corps Order 6110.10A, *Weight Control and Military Appearance,* Washington, D.C.: Department of the Navy, Headquarters United States Marine Corps, 1986.

Marine Corps Order 6100.10B, *Weight Control and Military Appearance,* enclosures 2 and 3, Washington, D.C.: Commandant of the Marine Corps, May 10, 1986.

Marine Corps Order 6100.13A CH-3, *Marine Corps Physical Fitness and Combat Fitness Tests (PFT/CFT),* Washington, D.C.: Department of the Navy, Headquarters United States Marine Corps, February 23, 2021. As of June 29, 2021:
https://www.marines.mil/Portals/1/Publications/MCO%206100.13A%20with%20CH-3.pdf

Marine Corps Order 6110.3, *Marine Corps Body Composition and Military Appearance Program*, Washington, D.C.: Department of the Navy, Headquarters U.S. Marine Corps, August 8, 2008.

Marine Corps Order 6110.3A CH-1 and Admin Ch, *Marine Corps Body Composition and Military Appearance Program*, Washington, D.C.: Department of the Navy, Headquarters United States Marine Corps, April 16, 2019. As of June 3, 2021:
https://www.fitness.marines.mil/Portals/211/documents/BCP%2020190502%20.pdf

Marine Corps Order P6100.12 CH-1, *Marine Corps Physical Fitness Test and Body Composition Program Manual*, Washington, D.C.: Department of the Navy, Headquarters U.S. Marine Corps, May 10, 2002.

McNulty, Peggy Anne Fisher, "Prevalence and Contributing Factors of Eating Disorder Behaviors in Active Duty Service Women in the Army, Navy, Air Force, and Marines," *Military Medicine*, Vol. 166, No. 1, January 2001, pp. 53–58.

MCO—*See* Marine Corps Order.

Merhej, Rita, "Dehydration and Cognition: An Understated Relation," *International Journal of Health Governance*, Vol. 24, No. 1, 2019, pp. 19–30.

Meyer, Nanna L., Jorunn Sundgot-Borgen, Timothy G. Lohman, Timothy R. Ackland, Arthur D. Stewart, Ronald J. Maughan, Suzanne Smith, and Wolfram Müller, "Body Composition for Health and Performance: A Survey of Body Composition Assessment Practice Carried Out by the Ad Hoc Research Working Group on Body Composition, Health and Performance Under the Auspices of the IOC Medical Commission," *British Journal of Sports Medicine*, Vol. 47, No. 16, 2013, pp. 1044–1053.

Navy Marine Corps 3500.7C, *Artillery Training and Readiness Manual*, Washington, D.C.: Department of the Navy, Headquarters United States Marine Corps, October 29, 2018. As of June 3, 2021:
https://www.marines.mil/Portals/1/Publications/NAVMC%203500.7C%20Artillery%20T-R%20Manual.pdf?ver=2020-04-21-123905-510

Nazem, Taraneh Gharib, and Kathryn E. Ackerman, "The Female Athlete Triad," *Sports Health*, Vol. 4, No. 4, July 2012.

O'Brien, Katie M., Denis R. Whelan, Dale P. Sandler, Janet E. Hall, and Clarice R. Weinberg, "Predictors and Long-Term Health Outcomes of Eating Disorders," *PLOS One*, Vol. 12, No. 7, July 2017, e0181104.

Office of Naval Operations Instruction 6110.1J, *Physical Readiness Program*, Washington, D.C.: Department of the Navy, Office of the Chief of Naval Operations, July 11, 2011. As of September 29, 2021:
https://www.netc.navy.mil/Portals/46/NSTC/OTCN/docs/OPNAVINST%206110.1J.pdf

Olson, Wyatt, "Heavier Female Soldiers Out-Perform Leaner Counterparts in Strength Tasks, Study Finds," *Military.com*, March 4, 2020. As of June 3, 2021: https://www.military.com/daily-news/2020/03/04/heavier-female-soldiers-out-perform-leaner-counterparts-strength-tasks-study-finds.html

OrthoInfo, "Female Athlete Triad: Problems Caused by Extreme Exercise and Dieting," webpage, August 2020. As of September 24, 2021: https://orthoinfo.aaos.org/en/diseases--conditions/female-athlete-triad-problems-caused-by-extreme-exercise-and-dieting

Pawlyk, Oriana, "Air Force Becomes First Service to Ditch the Hated Tape Test for Good," *Military.com*, December 8, 2020. As of June 21, 2021: https://www.military.com/daily-news/2020/12/08/air-force-becomes-first-service-ditch-hated-tape-test-good.html

Quade, E. S., *The Systems Approach to Public Policy*, Santa Monica, Calif.: RAND Corporation, P-4053, 1969. As of October 11, 2021: https://www.rand.org/pubs/papers/P4053.html

Reisman, Miriam, "PTSD Treatment for Veterans: What's Working, What's New, and What's Next," *Pharmacy and Therapeutics*, Vol. 41, No. 10, October 2016, pp. 623–634.

Roberto, Christina A., Laurel E. S. Mayer, Adam M. Brickman, Anna Barnes, Jordan Muraskin, Lok-Kin Yeung, Jason Steffener, Melissa Sy, Joy Hirsch, Yaakov Stern, and B. Timothy Walsh, "Brain Tissue Volume Changes Following Weight Gain in Adults with Anorexia Nervosa," *International Journal of Eating Disorders*, Vol. 44, No. 5, July 2011, pp. 406–411.

Rosen, James C., Nancy T. Silberg, and Janet Gross, "Eating Attitudes Test and Eating Disorders Inventory: Norms for Adolescent Girls and Boys," *Journal of Consulting and Clinical Psychology*, Vol. 56, No. 2, April 1988, pp. 305–308.

Rosen, Lionel W., and David O. Hough, "Pathogenic Weight-Control Behaviors of Female College Gymnasts," *Physician and Sportsmedicine*, Vol. 16, No. 9, September 1988, pp. 140–143.

Seck, Hope Hodge, "Volunteer Testing Begins in Marines' Groundbreaking Body Composition Study," *Military.com*, June 10, 2021. As of December 22, 2021: https://www.military.com/daily-news/2021/06/10/volunteer-testing-begins-marines-groundbreaking-body-composition-study.html

Schogol, Jeff, "The PFT and CFT Can Be Gender Neutral. Here's How," *Marine Times*, July 10, 2017. As of February 23, 2022: https://www.marinecorpstimes.com/off-duty/military-fitness/2017/07/10/the-pft-and-cft-can-be-gender-neutral-here-s-how

Seibert, Crescent A., *Demographic, Psychological, and Weight-Related Correlates of Weight Control Behaviors Among Active Duty Military Personnel*, thesis, Bethesda, Md.: Uniformed Services University of the Health Sciences, March 2007. As of September 24, 2021:
https://apps.dtic.mil/sti/pdfs/ADA476064.pdf

Sfera, Adonis, Michael Cummings, and Carolina Osorio, "Dehydration and Cognition in Geriatrics: A Hydromolecular Hypothesis," *Frontiers in Molecular Biosciences*, Vol. 3, article 18, May 2016.

Shufelt, Chrisandra L., Tina Torbati, and Erika Dutra, "Hypothalamic Amenorrhea and the Long-Term Health Consequences," *Seminars in Reproductive Medicine*, Vol. 35, No. 3, May 2017, pp. 256–262.

Silas, Sharon, *Department of Defense: Eating Disorders in the Military*, Washington, D.C.: U.S. Government Accountability Office, GAO-20-611R, August 7, 2020. As of June 3, 2021:
https://www.gao.gov/products/gao-20-611r

Sim, Leslie A., Donald E. McAlpine, Karen B. Grothe, Susan M. Himes, Richard G. Cockerill, and Matthew M. Clark, "Identification and Treatment of Eating Disorders in the Primary Care Setting," *Mayo Clinic Proceedings*, Vol. 85, No. 8, August 2010, pp. 746–751.

Sisbarro, Sharon, Kerry Hogan, Sara Kirstein, and Catherine Baniakas, "The DoD's Body Composition Standards Are Harming Female Service Members," *Military.com*, December 31, 2020. As of June 3, 20201:
https://www.military.com/daily-news/opinions/2020/12/31/dods-body-composition-standards-are-harming-female-service-members.html

Slane, Jennifer D., Michele D. Levine, Sonya Borrero, Kristin M. Mattocks, Amy D. Ozier, Norman Silliker, Harini Bathulapalli, Cynthia Brandt, and Sally G. Haskell, "Eating Behaviors: Prevalence, Psychiatric Comorbidity, and Associations with Body Mass Index Among Male and Female Iraq and Afghanistan Veterans," *Military Medicine*, Vol. 181, Nos. 11–12, November–December 2016, pp. e1650–e1656.

Stern, Carly, "Why BMI Is a Flawed Health Standard, Especially for People of Color," *Washington Post*, May 5, 2021.

Suhr, Julie A., Jessica Hall, Stephen M. Patterson, and Rebecca Tong Niinistö, "The Relation of Hydration Status to Cognitive Performance in Healthy Older Adults," *International Journal of Psychophysiology*, Vol. 53, No. 2, July 2004, pp. 121–125.

TeensHealth for Neumours, "Female Athlete Triad," webpage, July 2020. As of September 24, 2021:
https://kidshealth.org/en/teens/triad.html

Téllez, María José Arias, Francisco M. Acosta, Guillermo Sanchez-Delgado, Borja Martinez-Tellez, Victoria Muñoz-Hernández, Wendy D. Martinez-Avila, Pontus Henriksson, and Jonatan R. Ruiz, "Association of Neck Circumference with Anthropometric Indicators and Body Composition Measured by DXA in Young Spanish Adults," *Nutrients*, Vol. 12, No. 2, February 2020, p. 514.

Tompkins, Erin, *Obesity in the United States and Effects of Military Recruiting*, Washington, D.C.: Congressional Research Service, December 22, 2020. As of June 3, 2021:
https://fas.org/sgp/crs/natsec/IF11708.pdf

U.S. Department of Defense, *Study of the Military Services Physical Fitness*, Washington, D.C., April 3, 1981.

U.S. General Accounting Office, *Military Attrition: Better Data, Coupled with Policy Changes, Could Help the Services Reduce Early Separations*, report to the chairman and the ranking minority member, Subcommittee on Personnel, Committee on Armed Services, U.S. Senate, Washington, D.C., GAO/NSIAD-98-213, September 1998. As of October 11, 2021:
https://www.gao.gov/assets/nsiad-98-213.pdf

Wagner, Dale R., and Vivian H. Heyward, "Measures of Body Composition in Blacks and Whites: A Comparative Review," *American Journal of Clinical Nutrition*, Vol. 71, No. 6, June 2000, pp. 1392–1402.

Wells, Jonathan C. K., and M. S. Fewtrell, "Measuring Body Composition," *Archives of Disease in Childhood*, Vol. 91, No. 7, June 2006, pp. 612–617.

Winkie, Davis, "No More Tape Test? Army Study to Reevaluate Body Fat Program," *Army Times*, July 20, 2021. As of December 21, 2021:
https://www.armytimes.com/news/your-army/2021/07/20/no-more-tape-test-army-study-to-reevaluate-body-fat-program